THE COVERT NARCISSIST:

HOW TO IDENTIFY A NARCISSIST AND DEFEND YOURSELF FROM A TOXIC RELATIONSHIP, AVOIDING PHYSICAL AND PSYCHOLOGICAL ABUSE.

© **Copyright 2020 by Melanie Cohen - All rights reserved.**

The content contained within this book may not be reproduced, duplicated or transmitted without direct written permission from the author or the publisher.

Under no circumstances will any blame or legal responsibility be held against the publisher, or author, for any damages, reparation, or monetary loss due to the information contained within this book. Either directly or indirectly.

Legal Notice:

This book is copyright protected. This book is only for personal use. You cannot amend, distribute, sell, use, quote or paraphrase any part, or the content within this book, without the consent of the author or publisher.

Disclaimer Notice:

Please note the information contained within this document is for educational and entertainment purposes only. All effort has been executed to present accurate, up to date, and reliable, complete information. No warranties of any kind are declared or implied. Readers acknowledge that the author is not engaging in the rendering of legal, financial, medical or professional advice. The content within this book has been derived from various sources. Please consult a licensed professional before attempting any techniques outlined in this book.

By reading this document, the reader agrees that under no circumstances is the author responsible for any losses, direct or indirect, which are incurred as a result of the use of information contained within this document, including, but not limited to, — errors, omissions, or inaccuracies.

Table of Contents

Introduction 6

Chapter 1. Origins of a Narcissist 11

Chapter 2. Who Is A Hidden Narcissist? 17

Chapter 3. Am I a Narcissist? 21

Chapter 4. How One Becomes A Hidden Narcissist? 26

Chapter 5. How to Recognize, Detect, Or Unmask A Hidden Narcissist? 29

Chapter 6. How to Live with A Narcissist? 33

Chapter 7. Torque and Family dynamics with Narcissist Parents 39

Chapter 8. Differences Between Male and Female Narcissists 45

Chapter 9. Is a Hidden Narcissist Happy? 51

Chapter 10. What are the Secret Methods in Which Hidden Narcissists use Social media 56

Chapter 11. Exposing a Narcissist and Their Most Hidden Fears 61

Chapter 12. A Hidden Narcissist Suffers Internally? 66

Chapter 13. Benign and Malignant Narcissism (Overt and Covert) 69

Chapter 14. How your Life Changed when you Left a Narcissist 72

Chapter 15. Dangerous Covert Narcissist & Their Betrayals 78

Chapter 16. The Most Common Phrases of A Secret Narcissist 84

Chapter 17. Is A Narcissist Intelligent? 89

Chapter 18. What Are the Possible Cures for Narcissist? 94

Chapter 19. The Narcissist's Target 100

Chapter 20. Narcissists and Sex 105

Chapter 21. Three Types of Empathy 110

Chapter 22. Codependency and Narcissists 115

Chapter 23. The Narcissist and Psychological Games 121

Chapter 24. Narcissism and Addiction 125

Chapter 25. Narcissist Personalities 129

Chapter 26. The Narcissistic Scale 135

Chapter 27. Narcissism and Culture 138

Chapter 28. Dissecting the Workaholic Narcissist 144

Chapter 29. Things That Narcissistic Hate but Ordinary People Like .. 150

Conclusion 155

Introduction

Narcissists are highly manipulative people; thus, it could prove difficult to spot them, especially the older and more sophisticated ones. Throughout their lifetime, they master the art of manipulation, in other optimally abuse their victims without getting detected.

Their abuse pattern all have certain consistent traits – the idealization, devaluation, and discard of their romantic partners. However, there are different types of narcissists in terms of operation, and one such is the "Covert narcissist."

The covert narcissist is one of the toughest to spot because he operates from under the radar and is known to react in a passive-aggressive manner.

Covert narcissists create chaos in other people's lives and thrive from the resulting pain and anguish. One of their favorite pastimes is setting their victims up for failure and dish out some punishment when they ultimately fail. Sometimes, they intentionally make promises they know they won't keep, and when their victims react, they make it look like they're being victimized. Some even deny ever making any promise, resorting to gaslighting techniques to make their victims believe that they're losing their minds. It can lead to a dangerous result for the victim.

What Are the Characteristics of a Covert Narcissist?

Covert Narcissists Are Conflicted

Covert narcissists are conflicted, and it stems from the fact that they want to be worshipped. They are highly insecure, but the only thing they think about is themselves. By the way, it is effortless for them to trap their victims because they have mastered the art of using sob stories to suck in them. Covert narcissists have an eye for their potential victims, meaning they know how to detect people with empathy and conscience quickly.

They Manipulate People's Empathy

The truth about the situation is, whether the abuser is your lover, friend, or sibling, you're already aware of their issues. However, it is complicated to ignore them. Some of them may even contemplate suicide, making it more difficult for their victims to abandon them.

They do these things intentionally because they don't want to be held accountable for their actions. Some will use words like "since I was born, I've never felt this way about anybody."

Such emotional words give their victims a sense of responsibility and even boosts their impetus the more -they see it as a call to help them get back to their feet, even at their detriment.

Covert narcissists are all about their emotions. Thus, the victim's emotional wellbeing means nothing to them. As far as they are concerned, everything in life is a competition, and no matter what you're going through, it is nothing compared to what they've been through.

The Lie Sophisticated Lies

Covert narcissists have everything but love for others, and anything that challenges their sense of superiority is seen as a personal attack. They look down on everybody else, and when they encounter people they feel are better than them, they feel threatened and resort to talk-downs and insults. They always have an excuse for everything and are fond of rooting for the underdog because it makes them look better in public. Showing support for movements like feminism, gay rights, and other civil rights actions trick people into thinking that they have high morals; however, the opposite is the case.

It is usual for a covert narcissist to lie about his past, e.g., they'll lie about the famous people they used to hang out with or even the number of celebrities they've slept with; it is all lies.

Covert narcissists lack any sense of empathy or affection; however, they tend to watch TV a lot because they're trying to copy behaviors they see, e.g., compassion, love, and show of affection.

It is challenging for victims to escape from their covert abusers' clutches because they drain them physically, mentally, and psychologically.

Covert narcissists are like the most dangerous abusers because they use gaslighting and other forms of abuse to weaken their victims psychologically and mentally. It is often long after the narcissist has dumped the victim and moved on that the victim finally gets to realize that they've been grossly abused.

There is always hope, and as a victim, once you realize this, it is essential to seek help from the appropriate quarters to build your life all over again.

How Do I Deal with A Covert Narcissist?

At first, covert narcissists may seem charming and alluring, but after some time, you'll realize that they'll despise everything that comes out of your mouth, and even do things that'll make you question your self-worth and existence. At the office, they'll set you up to take the fall when things go wrong. They're damaged human beings, and as such, their mission is to degenerate people to a level where they won't even recognize themselves anymore.

Whenever you identify a covert narcissist, the best thing to do is to stay as far away as possible from them. However, if you must maintain an ongoing relationship with them, you must be mentally alert because, as you already know, they only exist to sabotage your efforts.

Irrespective of the narcissist position in your life, it is essential to maintain boundaries and protect yourself.

Desist from telling them intimate things about yourself and don't share your success stories with them, because they'll turn it around and deflate your excitement.

Here are the essential guides to keep in mind when dealing with covert narcissists;

Always Do It Their Way

Let a covert narcissist do what they want. Whether they choose to see a movie, buy a shirt, or even see a show, just let them do whatever they want.

Narcissists lead a sad and terrible life, but the most painful thing is that they know nothing about it. They think they're living a life of control and authority, but you know better; thus, allow peace to reign, and let them do whatever they choose to do.

Finally, it would help if you also remembered that you have the option of walking away and never looking back.

Always Put Yourself First

In your relationship with a covert narcissist, you have to consciously put yourself first, and still get what you need from them before considering any other thing.

Whatever thing you're doing with them, always conclude your part before you hand over control to them. It is essential because once they're in control, they will use their position to manipulate and exploit you. Remember, it is better to achieve small goals than to lose out on everything.

If you're related to the narcissist and you know you can't easily cut ties, you can nod your head, smile, and walk away whenever you guys meet. However, if you're dealing with someone in your workplace, you have to openly tackle them and make them understand that they are not better than you in any way.

Put the Spotlight on Them

Sometimes, instead of allowing have their way, you can choose to point out their wrong behaviors and confront them about it. As usual, they'll react by undermining you and your position, but if you're consistent, you might successfully crack them and make them look elsewhere for their narcissistic supply.

Understand that you cannot change who they are; however, you also have that you can make things extremely difficult for them.

Finally, as much as this has the potential of driving them away, for you to come out victorious, you must be willing to burn a lot of emotional energy in the process.

Stop Being Emphatic

Empathic people are highly vulnerable to covert narcissistic abuse because they are always willing to help out.

Narcissists are highly entitled to people with high expectations, and as such, they are always out to manipulate and deceive other people in other to achieve their motives. Thus, rather than feeling remorseful, you should stop caring about them and treat them the way they deserve to be treated.

You have to condition your mind to understand that they are responsible for their own lives, and no matter what you do, they'll never change. Thus, please do not waste your empathy on them!

Don't Deal with Them

Covert narcissists are incredibly deadly, and with techniques such as projection and gaslighting, they can ultimately damage your self-esteem and self-belief. Thus, rather than run the risk of being exposed to such covert attacks, the best thing to do is leave and quietly walk away.

Mind you; a typical narcissist is toxic, petty, and heartless – meaning they can do whatever it takes to discredit, shame, and destroy you. As human beings, they're even worthless to themselves, so, of what value are they in your life?

The primary assignment is to pull down others and make them feel less worthy of themselves as human beings. They magnify their victims' weaknesses and discredit their strengths; however, the most disturbing thing is that they love to see people in pain because it makes them feel strong.

If you're someone that appreciates and cherish your sanity, the most intelligent decision you can make in this situation is to cut ties and move on to more productive things.

Remember: if the person in question is family, do not fool yourself into believing that you can fix them. They are unfixable and irredeemable!

There are a lot of covert narcissists littered around the world and from different walks of life. These people are known to only care about their interests and public image. They are incredibly selfish individuals who ride on their high horses and always manipulate others for their gains. They cannot show empathy, and such, they bring some much pain and anguish in their victims' lives.

In the outside world, it is easy to spot them and deal with them, but when the narcissist is a family member, it becomes a different ball game. No matter where you find yourself, it is essential to set your boundary, keep your wits, and know your self-worth if you encounter any narcissist.

Chapter 1. Origins of a Narcissist

Let's look at the origin of the narcissist behavior and the disorder. Who first coined the term narcissist, and who put the condition in the psychology reference books? What famous psychologists worked in this field and who were and are famous narcissists today.

For this guide, we will be looking at historical or famous narcissists, whether they were diagnosed with Narcissistic Personality Disorder or not.

History of Narcissism

The behavior that we call narcissism has been around since the beginning of human history, but the term, the concept, and the disorder we call Narcissistic Personality Disorder is relatively new. In ordinary non-scientific or psychological terms, narcissism pursues personal gratification from egoistic vanity, from admiring yourself to the extreme. Narcissism is named after a young man in a Greek myth who fell in love with his image in a reflecting pool. His name was Narcissus. He eventually died from grieving over a love that did not exist.

In medieval times, this image had a lot of influence over the thinking. In Metamorphoses, Ovid retells the tale and alludes to the story. It supposedly influenced Shakespeare's Sonnets, and the term self-love was used for what Narcissus was feeling. Francis Bacon picked it up and used it in Pompey- as Cicero was said to call them, "lovers of themselves without rivals." Then came Byron early in the nineteenth century saying that self-love stings anything it stumbles on. Finally, Baudelaire talked about self-love as being like Narcissuses of fat-headedness.

Egotism became the new word for self-love in the mid-century, and lovers of self were now egotists – with Freud's use of the ego and the id. Narcissism then, as a concept, was coined and defined within the field of psychiatry, psychology, and psychoanalytic theory, by none other than Sigmund Freud.

Nacke had used the term as early as 1899, but he meant a sexual pervert. In 1911, Otto Rank picked up where Freud left off, identifying the word as vanity and self = admiration moving it back into the psychological realm, where it has stated within Narcissistic Personality Disorder.

Still, no one had more influence on the use of the term and the concept's psychology than Sigmund Freud. The year was 1914, and the essay was on narcissism, where Freud introduced the idea and used the word. By 1968 the American Psychiatric Association included the Narcissistic Personality Disorder in its Diagnostic and Statistical Manual of Mental Disorders associated with megalomania.

So, for a long time, NPD and Megalomania were considered to be the same thing. They are not as we have also recently referenced; all megalomaniacs are narcissists. Not all narcissists are megalomaniacs.

At the same time, narcissism has been defined as a social or cultural issue, more in the sociological study than psychological. It is because you can be a narcissist and not have Narcissistic Personality Disorder. You will find it listed among the three dark triadic personality traits of psychopathy, narcissism, and Machiavellianism. One factor in trait theory is self-report inventories like MCMI – the Million Clinical Multiaxial Inventory. From the outset, narcissism has been considered a problem for individuals and social groups. It was the end of the nineteenth century, and the term became a regular part of the language. The time is used in analytical writing more than anywhere else and perhaps more than any other word.

Just like with anything else, as time goes on, the meaning of words changes. It has happened somewhat with narcissism too. Today, the world has come to mean anything on a continuum from healthy self-love to a pathological sense of self.

In the Beginning

Sigmund Freud coined the scientific term and the disorder. He talked it in terms of a history of megalomania that was infantile according to his theory. He believed that as the person developed, they grew from egocentric to social in their orientations.

Others who felt megalomania was normal for children included Edmund Bergler, Otto Fenichel, and more. In the early 20th century, a new theory came into being, object relations theory. These modern theorists saw a defense mechanism in megalomania that would allow for therapy. At the same time, Freud saw megalomania as a problem for psychoanalysis. Some psychologists and psychiatrists saw megalomania as a part of the average growth and developmental pattern of a child, while others like Kemberg saw it as pathological. The popular culture also considers megalomania and narcissism to be the same thing.

Once the concept was set loose into the culture, it blossomed. Megalomania was seen in popular terminology, novels, and movies to mean a very self-centered, uncaring individual. Just one example is the character played by Nichole Kidman in "To Die For." She wants what she wants, and she will do anything to get it, including murder her husband. Those who saw the film rated this character a 9 or 10 with a prototypical Narcissistic Personality Disorder person as a 10.

Some others in the field did not see NPD as a separate personality disorder but as one part of the continuum of personality disorders. Alarcon and Sarabia, writing on this, claimed that NPD was not sociologically inconsistent, and more research needed to be done to consider it a dominant trait.

Yet the concept of narcissism was so central to Freud's thinking and his concept of psychotherapy. He considered narcissism to be a necessary development stage in growing from childhood to adulthood. In his work, he separated narcissism into Primary and Secondary Narcissism.

Primary Narcissism

In primary narcissism is the "desire and energy that drives our instinct to survive." For Freud, this included narcissism as more normal than it had been thought, just a part of growing and developing. Freud claimed that narcissism complemented "the egoism of the instinct of self-preservation." What was meant by this was we are born without ego or a sense of ourselves as separate individuals. Then we develop the ego and primary narcissism until society intrudes with its norms and standards to insist that we create an ideal ego – or move away from primary narcissism. The ego should aspire to a perfect self, one that can move to cathect objects. Freud defined the ego libido like that which is directed only toward oneself. Object-libido is directed toward other people or other items that are outside of the self.

Secondary Narcissism

Secondary narcissism occurs when the self-moves away from those objects and people outside of themselves, especially their mother. It leads the self toward the possibility of megalomania. Secondary narcissism, which is not healthy, is imposed upon primary narcissism, which is beneficial. Both types of narcissism develop in the ordinary course of human growth, but transitions can lead to Narcissistic Personality Disorder when you become an adult.

Freud believed the self/ego had only a certain amount of energy, and if it were turned toward objects or people outside itself, then there would not be any left for narcissism. As people develop, they move away from primary narcissism to giving their love to others instead of keeping it for themselves.

It is a healthy development, and the more love received in return, the less likely the person is to become pathologically narcissistic. To care for someone else is to transfer the ego-libido to an object-libido by giving away one's self-love. If this love is not returned or disrupted, then the individual's personality balance is upset and the potential for a psychological upset.

Beyond Freud

Following this, Karen Horney presented a very different view of narcissism than that put forward by mainstream psychoanalytic theorists such as Kohut and Freud. Her idea of selfishness did not include primary narcissism but rather posited that narcissism came about from the kind of early environment that poisoned the child's ability to develop a healthy personality. Karen Horney believed that narcissism is not inherent in human nature.

Then along comes Heinz Kohut and his theory that a child is only fantasizing about having ideal parents and a grandiose self. He theorized that we all believed in perfection in ourselves and anything we participated in. This belief in the glorious self becomes healthy self-esteem, and the child's core values come from idealizing the parents. Kohut believed that if the child is then traumatized, the child reverts to the most primitive version of the narcissistic self. That version then remains primary for that person as they grow to adulthood. It becomes a Narcissistic Personality Disorder. The child does not relate to the external object but rather unites with their idealized self-object.

He also believed that you would or could get beyond pathological narcissism either through analysis or life experiences. He felt if you could get beyond the pathology, you could develop ambition, ideals, and resilience for good.

Then comes Otto Kornberg, who thought narcissism was simply the self-played role in regulating one's self-esteem. He thought infantile narcissism was normal as long as the child was exposed to the affirmation of self and "acquisition of desirable and appealing objects." These objects would then become a part of the individuals' mature and healthy self-esteem. Narcissism becomes pathological if infantile narcissism does not develop into healthy self-esteem for whatever reason.

Other vital theorists since Freud include Melanie Klein, Herbert Rosenfeld, D.W. Winnicott, and the French with Lacan, Bela Grumberger, and Andre Green.

Narcissistic Personality Disorder Today

Today the DSM-IV contains Narcissistic Personality Disorder, but there have been requests to remove it and submerge the condition into the antagonism personality type domain. NPD it the "it" disorder of the twenty-first century. How will history remember our foray into this condition? There are now subtypes of narcissism that were not around before. Those are antisocial, prosocial, idealizing, mirroring, malignant, vulnerable, grandiose, and exhibitionist.

NPD is a diagnosis that becomes more common every day. Is it just trendy, or is it for some reason more prevalent? Do we truly have a "Culture of Narcissism" as Christopher Lasch proposed in his 1979 book by the same name? He believes that NPD has become the typical way of living in American culture today.

Chapter 2. Who Is A Hidden Narcissist?

The narcissist is the perfect pretender. She is a wolf in sheep's clothing. Scratch that — she is Mystique from the X-Men. The narcissist understands that her true self is unacceptable. Because of this, the narcissist does their best to create a false persona. They put a lot more energy into developing this ideal character than Quentin Tarantino puts into writing his characters. The narcissist is the ultimate method actor — with the ability to completely abandon one character or mask in favor of another in a heartbeat. Why is this so? Remember, the narcissist is a predator. The last thing a predator need is for its prey to recognize it when it crouches, ready to kill.

The Narcissist's Vibe

Narcissists are both similar to and different from each other. At their very core, they are pretty much the same thing and have the same desire — being the center of attention and dominating everything and everyone. They all do this by merely manipulating others into giving them the reactions they want. However, this is where the similarities end. All narcissists live in different situations, and so they adapt accordingly. Malignant narcissists are arrogant; they brag a lot; they are vain, cocky, and entitled. They are also utterly glorious, and it's hard to miss their arrogance in the way they carry themselves, the way they dress, the way they talk.

Not all narcissists are this way, though. Some are a far cry from all those adjectives I described the toxic narcissist with. Some narcissists are skilled at keeping all that haughtiness tightly sealed and under wraps, cloaked with faux modesty. They only ever let their freak flag fly when they're with those who are close to them.

Narcissists are adept at adapting to their surroundings. If a narcissist would ordinarily be flamboyant, gregarious, and loud in the city, he would tone it down in the smaller towns where such behavior is frowned upon. The narcissist knows when it's time to be all glorious — when it matters that they pass themselves off as necessary — and when it's time to be "humble" — so everyone marvels at how remarkably modest he is.

Look a Little Closer

It might seem that because the narcissist is so adaptable, it would be hard to detect her. But you can. All you need to do is look a little bit closer. Grandiosity is not an easy thing to hide, no matter how subtle the narcissist is about it. You can detect t in the way they relate with others. There's that barely palpable aura of them feeling above it all, and better than you. There's a hint of judgmental in the way they talk with others. It's there in the presumptions they have about what they feel ought to be done, as they present their opinions as mere suggestions, and touched up with that false modesty and humility. Then there's the bragging. It always creeps in somehow.

Not all narcs are elegantly dressed, have a house in the Hamptons, a movie in the works, and act out when their trailer is not set just so. Some narcissists present themselves as regular people. They dress. They don't seem the least bit vain and don't say too much.

Then others talk a lot — and you'll usually find these types working as preachers or politicians. They like to show themselves off as holier-than-thou, the last righteous man or woman in a morally bankrupt world, the one politician who wants to sacrifice himself for the good of all others. You can also find this kind being CEOs admired by all. A few others are dictators, greatly feared. The point to take away from all this is that you can't assume just because someone "fits the profile" — whatever that profile is in your head — they are a narcissist.

Image is Everything

The narcissist does not mess about when it comes to his appearance. He adapts to whatever the situation or environment requires of him. When he needs attention, he knows just how to be and what to wear to stand out. When it's time to get approval for something, he knows the perfect way to blend right in with the crowd.

The narcissist is not two-faced. She has many faces. She's different when she's at home and different when she's at work. She's different when she's with her colleagues, and different when she's with her family. She's one way when you're dating her, and she's another way entirely when you're married. It's almost as if a narcissist has multiple personas. You never be sure when it comes to the narcissist. You can bank on one thing, though — his image is the complete opposite of who he is.

Astute Observers

The narcissist pays special attention to the way humans behave, both as individuals and in group settings. They understand the dynamics of human interaction better than the average person. It's natural for human beings to figure out how to gain approval and acceptance, and then adopt that behavior. The narcissist knows this.

How she takes advantage of this tendency in humans is by being mercurial. She blows hot, then cold, then not at all. These arbitrary and random behavior keeps the people around her in a state of suspense, uncertainty, and insecurity. The people around her become afraid of saying or doing anything, fearing that it might be the wrong thing. And when you're around her, no matter what you say or do, it's never right.

As far as the narcissist is concerned, they and they alone deserve all the attention. If they can't get it for themselves, then there's going to be trouble. Usually, a narcissist will not get that much attention at home. That's because everyone at home already knows them for who they are. What does the narcissist do then? He must seek some attention somewhere by either being aggressive and causing fights, running his mouth, or generally being a nuisance.

The first-time psychiatry touched on the subject of narcissism; it was recorded as having the God Complex. That's basically when someone thinks they're a god and need to be worshipped accordingly. Said someone is typically a narcissist.

The narcissist is a god unto himself, and unto you, as far as he is concerned. You only exist because he says you exist. Your sole purpose is to amuse him — regardless of what that might mean for you. You're here for him, and no one and nothing else. Not even yourself. You're all about his interests, and if you aren't, there will be hell to pay. You owe him your very breath. He owns you - like furniture or something.

Because the narcissist owns you, they have the divine right to pass judgment on you. As their thing, they get to decide what your worth is if at all it exists. They can end you, and they can give your life. It all depends on what games they feel like playing at each point in time.

Do you ever judge a god? Of course not! So how dare you judge a narcissist? It's not even possible; they are perfect; they have no flaws and make no mistakes. On account of who they are, they're the good guy. It doesn't make any difference what they say or does. They are always the good guy. Everything they do is golden, because, duh, it's a narcissist! However, if anyone else did the same thing, then that person is very much in the wrong and should be judged and punished for it.

The narcissist is the king of double standards. As a god, he does not need to adhere to the standards he has so graciously set for others to follow. He is above it all. A narcissist can do whatever he wants to, and all would be just peachy, because, hey, he is a god, anyway. Gods can do whatever they want and get away with it. If they made you, then they can unmake you. Pretty simple. On account of his being god, there is absolutely no reason for the narcissist to trouble himself following the rules he set for you, puny mortal.

Know what else you can liken to this "God Complex" that the narcissist suffers from? I'll give you some hints. Who do you know who is super important, and for whom others exist to serve, no matter the cost? Who do you know who is owed the whole world and a couple of bank vaults as well? Who do you know should be given attention every time they so much as open their mouths? Babies. Yes, your narcissists — even the oh-so-terrifying malignant narc — are little more than babies.

Chapter 3. Am I a Narcissist?

Narcissistic tendencies are always problematic, but there are times when it is worse than others. A 'healthy' dose of narcissism can be beneficial to you. It is defined as having self-esteem while still maintaining a connection to others. It is self-love without being detrimental to others. However, this isn't always the case. Sometimes the narcissistic tendencies are extreme and need some profound changes to be made. If this is something you fear might be affecting you or someone in your life, please read on for more information.

Sociopath

A sociopath is someone who is usually defined by a lack of empathy. Someone with an antisocial personality is often seen as a sociopath as they do not interact with others because people without this form of narcissism do. They're known for being very charming and likable, but this is all a façade. Underneath all of that superficial falseness, they're calculating and have controlling behavior.

Here is a list of an indication to look out for:

- Being deceitful and lying. For example, they might con others and feel no remorse or use an alias to hide or what they're doing.
- An inability to follow social norms. They may act in inappropriate ways, from speaking out of turn to breaking the law.
- Overly assertive or aggressive behavior. It may be prone to getting into physical fights.
- An absence of empathy for others' feelings, even if they are responsible for those feelings.

- A display of very shallow feelings
- Impulsive behavior can hinder planning for the future.
- Lack of concern for others' safety.
- Irresponsibility that drives inconsistent behavior
- Taking part in reckless behavior, such as stealing, promiscuity, and taking uncalculated risks.

This behavior is worrying because it can lead to abusive relationships, aggression, and even violence. The longer that people allow it to continue, the worse it will get. The further a sociopath will push the boundaries to see what they can get away with. It needs to be allocated right away to protect everyone who comes into contact with this person. If you happen to be positive with this list or know someone who shows no remorse for their actions, no matter what they've done, and they also don't recognize that they have something they need to change about themselves, then they might be a narcissistic sociopath. Studies have shown this even often emanates from neglecting parents, sociopathic parents, or traumatic, abusive events. It can best be treated with a medical professional's help, and it's usually done via therapy.

Psychopath

Before this study, it has always been believed that psychopaths lack emotions and empathy, but it's more that they don't consider what will happen eventually. It all makes sense when the number of criminals who display these tendencies. Still, another research project found that fully functioning, successful adults with high-flying careers also show the same brain activity as a psychopath.

Here are some signs you can detect a psychopath:
- Superficial charm to lure people in at first.
- Ignoring huge problems with a non-committal attitude
- An inflated sense of self.
- A need for stimulation from extreme activities
- Lying, conning, manipulating.
- Lack of guilt even when pain is caused.
- Shallow feelings, no depth of emotions

- No empathy.
- Lacking control, promiscuous behavior, other behavioral issues
- Impulsive, irresponsible, no long-term goals.
- A tendency towards criminal activity.

The earlier these tendencies are spotted, the more chance you can help someone or even your own-self. By letting these traits to continue, you are letting it get worse. Psychopaths will use weaknesses against every victim to get what they want. The right thing you can do for yourself is to extract yourself from the situation, if possible before you get harmed. If doing this isn't possible, then you need some medical help for your loved one.

Narcopath

A narcopath is a narcissist-sociopath mix and is considered the worst type. Someone with an inflated sense of how important they are, as well as a constant need for praise and admiration – which already sounds exhausting! Relationships with them can be addictive, but draining as the person with a narcopath will never win.

Here is an excellent checklist for identifying whether you are involved with a narcopath:

- Things move fast – really fast! Instead of getting to know you, a narcopath will immediately make you feel like you've found your soul mate.
- The compliments – at first, they might feel nice, but after a while, you might realize that they're generic and maybe a bit staged.
- Flattery comes in the form of comparisons. It is especially bad if it links to an ex. Even if you come out on top, that won't last.
- You have strong chemistry. The passion is off the charts, but not much else is good.
- Hollow eyes that lead to nothing. It's all an act.
- The conversation always swivels back to themselves.
- A checkered relationship history is a sign of things to come.
- The silent treatment is standard.

It is another severe form of narcissism that can lead to abuse and violence if left untreated. It isn't always easy to confront someone who behaves in such a way, but doing so can lead to a happier future for the perpetrator and everyone in their life. Some therapy, especially cognitive behavioral therapy, can help with this.

The red flags of manipulation include:

- Your words being used against you.
- They offer you help, but their support leaves you confused and unhappy.
- They say shocking things, then claim that you misunderstood them.
- A lot of what they do is designed to make you feel guilt and shame.
- You question your sanity.
- Love and affection are withdrawn once you don't obey them.
- You fear losing that person, no matter what they do.
- You always feel like you fall short of expectations.
- You have been on eggshells with that person.
- You feel isolated by them.

If you feel any of these things happening in your life, you need to start thinking about taking some serious action. Read on for ways to help yourself and the narcissism sufferer.

It's seen as so beneficial that we even have some tips to help you gain some narcissism in your life to boost confidence when times are tough:

- Establish your own identity; don't worry what others expect of you.
- Feel proud when you reach your goals.
- Give yourself affirmations.
- Consider what you like about yourself.
- Care for yourself.
- Be kind to yourself, but also others.
- Allow yourself to have imperfections.

- When you feel bad, please do something to change it.
- Share in the success of others.

Chapter 4. How One Becomes A Hidden Narcissist?

Narcissism usually develops in early childhood. It seems the emotional trauma responsible for narcissism occurs around the age of a toddler; hence the narcissist's ability to handle emotions gets stuck at that level of mental development. That explains their dangerous emotional immaturity.

We all get exposed to trauma during the early stages of our development. It's only inevitable. Trauma can result from as simple as not being picked up by our parent as a baby or being fed against our will. It could also result from something more severe, as our mother left us at the kindergarten for the first time, causing a long-lasting fear of separation. Our parents fighting and screaming at each other in our presence can leave their imprints on our subconscious mind, too. So, what kind of trauma produces a narcissist?

Growing up with an overbearing and completely neglectful parent can warp a child's mind and cause them to be narcissistic adults eventually in life. A parent can be overpowering when it comes to a child's school performance and neglectful when it comes to a child's emotional needs. The trauma of a narcissist is the perceived lack of control. The inability to acknowledge their own emotions makes a narcissist extremely uncomfortable. Admitting one "wrong" thing about themselves would make them feel as though everything is wrong. So, every abusive and manipulative action they take only serves one purpose: to feel in control. The root of their toxic behavior towards you has nothing to do with you; it has everything to do with them. If you play close attention to their accusations, you will see that they project their behavior, fears, and doubts on you. A narcissist may often lie, yet accuse you of lying all the time, no matter how much proof you present that they are wrong. They may feel as if everyone is out to get them and always get the short end of the stick, so they project their subconscious beliefs on you by accusing you of plotting schemes against them every time there is a simple misunderstanding.

You must keep in mind that narcissists never truly learned how to express and process their emotions. Their parents may have been overly protective and proud of them – but only when they fulfilled their parents' expectations. One could try to do some research about the past of the narcissist in question. Though it usually is challenging to get a clear picture. It's tough to find the truth about a narcissist, especially when their parents admit to not having been able to handle their child.

In many cases, one or both of their parents may display some narcissistic traits, too. But, that doesn't mean that the kids of a narcissist are bound to become narcissistic as well.

It's not based on you to determine why the person that mistreated you has become who they are today, and it also not necessary for your recovery process. However, what is needed for your recovery process is that you are aware that it's not your fault in any way that they are a narcissist, and with that, you are not responsible for their chronic toxicity.

It can be an environmental cause that can lead to a forced image of perfection eventually in life. Another aspect is early childhood abuse. One way to deal with abuse is to see yourself as above it, too clean for it. Due to an abusive history, narcissism acts as a wall to prevent being hurt further in the future. Despite the several ways the disorder can be environmental, some believe that the trait can be hereditary. With genetics, though, seeing a specific behavioral feature can be difficult. Though it may seem genetic, it is the way that parent or grandparent was raised that gives them the condition. It brings up the question of actual genetics. Science has yet to come to a clear conclusion on that, though.

Studies have not reached a definite conclusion, and with many different conditions, it is hard to see, which is environmental and genetic.

The majority of the cases of Narcissistic Personality Disorder, though, always points back to the parents who raised the child. Whether it is neglect, abuse, overprotection, rewarding for insignificance, Munchausen, or even the parent giving the child a hypochondriac disorder or a sense that they are superior, their behavior is usually created an early age. With a deep-seated basis and such a long time for growth, this makes the disorder even harder to overcome eventually in life. Changing someone's perspective of how they should see the world when they were raised and to see it differently can be a nearly impossible task. It also can cause more behavioral and personality issues. Taking away the one or only defense someone has constructed to deal with trauma can lead to an exposed and vulnerable feeling that can cause depression and anxiety. What happens then is the person goes from being narcissistic to high-risk Avoidant Personality Disorder, agoraphobia, social anxiety, self-harm, and even suicidal, or an intention of hurting others. People using narcissism to cover an abusive or traumatic childhood would have to be approached with the utmost care.

Even if the issues are genetic, there is no direct way to treat genetics over a learned behavior cycle. Hereditary behavior issues are something a species line has evolved to. Somehow that series of genetics has become to see itself as more significant than others. Whether this has to do with the biological mating habits or some protective reaction of the line is part of who they are. Just as someone is likely to have a stronger inclination to be a leader or one who helps people for a living, being someone who sees themselves as above others will already be in their head from early childhood. As with learned behavior, this comes from one or both parents. If the parent(s) has the same genetic disposition, they will raise the child with that frame of mind; once again, the person is locked in a cycle. Being both genetically superior and raised to believe that they are so will be the prime persona of the person, which is not easy to change.

Chapter 5. How to Recognize, Detect, Or Unmask A Hidden Narcissist?

Identifying a narcissistic person can be comfortable in certain circumstances but very difficult in others. Those who are overtly narcissistic are naturally easier to remember. They are often loud, they hog all the attention, and they always want people to surround them. The covert narcissists can be challenging to identify because although they have the same common traits of seeking attention and have an equally inflated sense of self- importance, the manifestations are quite different.

You will not find a covert narcissist immediately bursting into a rage the moment you defy them. They will simper in favor in private, and their anger is usually manifested when you least expect it. Once the harm is done, they will again go back to their usual self, leaving the victim with the idea that it was all their imagination, and it was just an off-hand thing to have happened.

The difficulty of identifying a covert narcissist makes it all the more difficult to deal with them. It is not easy to understand that narcissistic behavior is not always associated with NPD or Narcissistic Personality Disorder, which is a stable behavioral pattern and involves cognitive, emotional, and interpersonal patterns.

Hence, when you meet a narcissistic person, you have no idea of knowing which kind of narcissism the person is afflicted with and

whether it is a personality disorder which can also be tackled with professional help. But what to do is to try and identify whether he or she is a narcissist at all and then get the person the help he or she needs.
A person who is a narcissist will have some triggers that will alert you about his personality. Here are some of the signs to look out for:
Does he often talk down to you? A narcissist will always talk down to you. For a covert narcissist, this is difficult to identify at first, but you will often find that he or she taking a condescending tone while speaking to you. On the off chance that he listens to what you have to say, he will give off the impression that it is not because the narcissist is genuinely interested in your opinion but that he is just humoring you. When this keeps on happening time, and again, there are high chances of being a narcissist.

Does he dismiss whatever you say or you plan? A narcissist will almost always dismiss your plans and ideas. In some cases, it happens immediately, as with an overt narcissist. In the case of a covert narcissist, it could happen more slowly. He or she will give off the impression of thinking about whatever you have had to say, but in the end, he will always dismiss your idea. If you have planned, they will manage to find some flaw in it and will subtly remark how you cannot get anything right unless they step up to help you out.

Is he disrespectful of you in public? A narcissist will often be rude to you in public. It is because narcissists resent their partners getting any attention over them. So, the moment that starts happening, they will do something to hurt your self-confidence, and by the time you go out of the room to gather your thoughts and make things easier for yourself, he or she would have managed to hog all the limelight. He or she will harp on how you could not be as successful as you were unless they helped you out or maybe, your success was a fluke, and you did not deserve it at all.

Will he often try to superimpose his ideas over yours? A narcissist will always try to superimpose his or her images over yours. The moment you have to say something, they will try to show they can do it better. If you try to do something, they will show it can be done better and only done their way. Your ideas will always be shot down, no matter how best you try to present them.

Does he become aloof and distant the moment you deny him? Narcissists can become very distant and cold in a matter of minutes. One moment they are all friendly and happy, talking to everyone and basking in the limelight. The moment you say or do anything that is not in keeping with what they wanted to hear, they can shut off. It's like not getting their favorite drink when they ordered it. While overt narcissists will stomp in rage and break into an outburst, covert narcissists are more likely to give you the silent treatment, and unless you make up for it to them, they will refuse to come out of their shells.

Is he always showing off his achievements to others? While it is alright to speak of one's success from time to time and seeking validation from others is a typical human trait, a narcissist will keep on doing this all the time. They will always speak of their achievements, sometimes even at the cost of others. At times, narcissism can make a person an over-achiever but truly propel them to achieve something great in life, but they do it without humility even if they do so.

Will, he always says that others need improvement, and he is perfect? For a narcissist, everything that he or she does is perfect. If anything goes wrong, it is because of someone else on the team in the workplace, or it was the wife's or the children's fault at home. They are perfect and need no improvement whatsoever. If anyone does manage to find fault with them, it is the other person's problem and not theirs.

Does he always try to outdo others? Narcissists will always try to beat others without giving others their dues, which could lead to very unhealthy competition at the workplace or cause relationship issues at home. It is alright to have some game from time to time, as it keeps the other person motivated, but too much can lead to friction. With narcissists, there is always the chance of conflict because of their habit of taking all the credit.

Do they never acknowledge their mistake? Narcissists will rarely admit their mistakes. They are stubborn, and they will refuse to see anything is wrong with them. Asking for an apology is beneath them, and they will make the other person feel inferior by continually pointing out their mistakes in turn.

For the victims of narcissistic abuse, it is challenging to keep up with these mood swings, and life becomes a constant struggle in trying to find out what the narcissist wants. If this happens to go on for long durations, it could lead to very traumatizing life experiences for narcissistic abuse victims.

If you feel that anyone you know at work or your partner manifests the signs mentioned above and symptoms, you suggest therapy. At times, therapy can help with a narcissistic attitude. If the problem is more profound and has become a deep-rooted psychological problem, it could be way more challenging to rein in the personality's narcissistic side. However, therapy is always the right place to start, and it provides an insight into the extent of the problem. Not all narcissists are unmanageable- at times, they manifest such behavior because they feel they would be left behind if they do not always develop ways to project themselves and promote themselves to others.

Once they feel seen and heard and start believing there are people around who are ready to listen to them, then the narcissistic behavior could go down over time. Residues of narcissistic traits will always be there in a narcissist. Still, it becomes easier to live with the person if both the parties involved have a clear understanding of the condition, and they are also willing to consider what is at stake if they choose to go different paths.

Narcissists can give you a hard time, but the good thing is that unlike other conditions, their behavior can be regulated unless the person also has other traits that turn them violent. If the state is only emotional, then with some help, you could still choose to have a long life with a narcissist partner.

However, it is a fact that there will always be some sacrifices to be made on the partner's behalf, and it is essential to understand one's limit to get out of a lifetime of trauma. However, by setting some boundaries for yourself, you could find a way of co-living with a narcissist and eventually find a middle-ground conducive to both.

Chapter 6. How to Live with A Narcissist?

Occasionally, it might not be possible to leave the narcissist. A parent might recognize narcissistic traits in an adult child, but severing ties with the child might not be an option to the parent. A spouse might not be willing to leave the narcissistic partner for religious or financial reasons. A child may realize the parent is a narcissist but may not have the heart to cut the parent out of the child's life. In all the situations mentioned here, severing ties with the narcissist isn't an option.

How can anyone learn to put with all the narcissistic traits of an individual without losing their sanity? How can you tolerate the narcissist's manipulative, controlling, and even annoying ways? Well, here are a couple of ideas that will come in handy while living with a narcissist.

Studying Them

You need to learn the narcissist, not from the perspective of a loved one, but from as an outsider. If you cannot do this, then none of the other tips talked in this part will work. When you objectively start studying the narcissist, you will better learn how to detach yourself mentally and emotionally. If you can analyze a narcissist's behavior dispassionately, it will give you the clarity you need to restore your emotional balance.

Call Out

Most narcissists tend to be immensely proud of their narcissism and think of it as a positive personality trait. You must call out the narcissist for their narcissistic ways. It will only work if the narcissist also values and cherishes the relationship you share. If that's the case, then use a measured and non-sarcastic tone to tell the narcissist that their narcissism is showing.

Cycle of Abuse

The narcissistic cycle of abuse is unique, and there are four steps involved. The stages are to feel threatened, abuse others, become the victim, and feel empowered. A narcissist goes through all these stages quite regularly. Learn to identify the different behaviors or words the narcissist uses in each of these stages. Once you can identify each of these steps, it is easier to break the cycle.

Tactics of Abuse

Narcissists tend to be creatures of habit. If narcissists realize that a specific tactic of abuse works, they will keep repeating it. A person can be subjected to seven types of abuse: physical, emotional, verbal, financial, spiritual, sexual, and mental. Some common tactics used by narcissists include coercion, gaslighting, love bombarding, aggression, threats, twisting the facts, and shifting the guilt. Make a note of all the different tactics the narcissist uses and come up with ways in which you can counter those tactics.

Play A Game

Narcissists tend to use their charm to attract others by asking them questions about the other person. However, they seldom listen to the answers and instead use it to talk about themselves. Instead of getting irritated when they do this, you can try this: Play a game to see how quickly they change the topics and increase this time with every conversation. Try to get the narcissist to stick to a subject for longer with each conversation you have.

Be Wary of Surprises

Like the Trojan horse as a cautionary tale while dealing with narcissists. The Greek army wanted to invade Troy's city without being detected, and they filled a giant wooden horse with gifts and a hidden army. When the horse was under control inside the city, the Greek army overtook the city. Every contribution that you receive from a narcissist must be treated with a little caution.

Feed Their Ego

A narcissist needs a lot of attention, affection, praise, and adoration to thrive. So, by complimenting him and feeding his fragile ego, you can easily handle living with a narcissist. You must be prepared to keep feeding his ego; if not, be ready to deal with his tantrums. If leaving the narcissist is not an option for you, you will need to get used to it. A couple of simple compliments can go a long way while trying to deal with a narcissist. It is not manipulation. Instead, it is about understanding his personality disorder and using it to help smooth things out.

Manage Your Expectations

Narcissists lack empathy. They certainly expect sympathy from others, but will seldom reciprocate. This absence of empathy makes it difficult for a narcissist to develop close and intimate bonds with others. It would help if you learned to accept and make peace with this. So, stop seeking empathy or compassion from the narcissist and instead try to manage your expectations.

Insecurities

Narcissists are often riddled with several insecurities. If you use their insecurities as retaliation, the narcissists will only get offended and become too defensive. Instead, it would help if you worked on supporting the narcissists to protect their insecurities and vulnerabilities.

Boundaries Matter

If you want to avoid the blame game, you must establish certain boundaries. It is unlikely that narcissists will apologize for their mistakes, but they will expect this humility from you. They can also exaggerate the other's wrongs to reduce the intensity of their own. Instead, it is time to place every mistake in context, don't apologize to maintain peace, and don't bother shifting the blame onto the narcissist. Prevent yourself from stooping to their level while handling them.

Embarrassment

Nothing triggers a narcissist as public humiliation does. Being publicly humiliated is the ultimate act of transgression for a narcissist. If the narcissist does something which can lead to public embarrassment, try to stand by his side. Narcissists value loyalty, especially when shown in times of their shame. Apart from this, try not to subject the narcissist to any public humiliation.

Seek Good

A personality disorder doesn't make anyone evil; it merely distorts the person's perception of reality. Sometimes, it is hard to find any good in the narcissist. A little practice will help while trying to seek any interest in the narcissist. Whenever you experience any negative feeling bubbling up about the narcissist, try to replace it with something positive.

You must evaluate things for yourself whether you want the narcissist in your life or not. If yes, you need to develop a lot of patience and become immune to his negative traits.

Get your Life Back on Track

It is essential to note that narcissists are not individuals who switch into their disorder while under stress. Narcissism is referred to as a personality disorder for this reason. It is who they are at all times and not just at some times. Your traits of compassion, empathy, and forgiveness are the ones the narcissistic partner used against you. In this part, you will learn about specific things you can do to kickstart the process of recovery and get your life back on track.

Set Boundaries

You need to set boundaries. If you want the process of healing to begin, you must establish a protective wall around yourself. Memories related to the narcissist and the relationship will undoubtedly trigger pain and other unpleasant emotions that, in turn, will slow down your progress. So, cut off all ties with the narcissist. You can block that individual on social media, your phone, and even an email list. Throw all the things that will remember you of the narcissist. It is time to remove all traces of connection with the narcissist.

Eliminate All Toxicity

It is time to get all this toxicity out of your system so you can start thinking once again. The best idea is to begin externalizing it. You can start maintaining a journal to write about what you have been through, talk to those friends you trust, consult a therapist, or even join a support group. A support group is a great help because it will connect you with others who experienced all you did.

Acknowledgment

It would help if you acknowledged the narcissistic abuse you were subjected to in your past. It would help if you accepted that the narcissist was a toxic individual and tried to hurt you consciously and without remorse. Please understand that you were not only tricked and manipulate, but you were abused too. Your ability to endure pain was used against you, and with each cycle of abuse, the narcissist kept pushing your limits. The narcissist managed to get away with his acts by seeing the good in the narcissist and ignoring the warning signs springing up around you.

Realization

You must realize that some part of you knew that you were stuck in a toxic situation. However, you chose to silence that little voice in your head. Now it is time to take some responsibility, and you must rationally analyze what happened. Maybe you experienced a feeling that something was wrong during the initial phase of the relationship. Perhaps certain things the narcissists said didn't add up. A post-mortem analysis of the relationship is essential. Now you know that there were several red flags you chose to ignore, and it is time to look at such instances.

Self-inquiry

Surviving narcissistic abuse is your wake-up call! Your vulnerabilities make you susceptible to manipulation. If you no longer wish to be manipulated and want to prevent manipulation at all costs, you must discover your vulnerabilities. There are specific common vulnerabilities like the need for security, need to be loved, and acknowledgment. These vulnerabilities can enable manipulation if left unchecked.

Healing

If you want to heal yourself, you need to take a walk down your memory lane and revisit your childhood. It helps create a sense of cohesiveness and eliminates any unresolved issues while fostering a strong connection with your inner self. Your inner child was hurt because of narcissistic abuse. Your inner child needs your help to heal. Only when you reconnect with your inner child will you be able to understand the root of any fears and insecurities you harbor. No, it doesn't mean that you must start acting childish. Instead, it means it is time to connect with your childlike side. It is about re-establishing a connection with that part of your psyche that is pure and innocent. There are methods in which you can heal your inner child. You can start saying loving things to your inner child and treat him with consideration and love.

Focus

There are times when you feel like your past is drawing you in. The combination of cognitive discord and the trauma bond you shared with the narcissist is the reason for this. If you feel like this, it means that you are yet to understand and process some emotions. It is quintessential you keep working to overcome the abuse you were a victim of. Instead of letting your past rob your present, allocate some time for yourself where you can analyze your past.

Be Patient

You must be patient with yourself. You cannot hurry up and rush through the process of recovery. There will be times when you feel like you are staring at a bottomless pit of despair; you might get frustrated or might even feel quite depressed. Well, this merely means you need to concentrate on healing yourself.

Chapter 7. Torque and Family dynamics with Narcissist Parents

The way narcissist parents handle their children's relationships can be quite frustrating and often always affects their children's emotional needs. Growing up with such parents can be very lonely, draining, and exasperating.

During our childhood, the strongest bond and primary attachment we have is that we feel for our parents. When hungry, scared, tired, or ill, they are the first people we turn to.

The absence of this bond helps explain why relationships with narcissist parents are so disappointing. Our instincts prompt us to keep turning to our parents for care and understanding. The following are some of the difficulties of having a narcissist parent:

It Is Difficult to Communicate with Them

Narcissist parent has poor communication skills. Interacting with them is very frustrating; they make others feel like they have been shut down or shut out. They have a minimal range of attention when it comes to the interests of other people.

Interacting with emotionally immature people is usually one-sided. They are not interested in having reciprocal conversations; they hunger for exclusive attention and want everyone to show interest in what they are interested in. If they are no longer the center of attention, they find ways to bring back their attention.

They Stimulate Anger in their Children

Anger is an adaptive reaction to feelings of neglect, rejection, and abandonment. It is a sign of distress to unhealthy emotional situations. Feelings of anger or rage are perfectly normal reactions to personal injury.

In some cases, the children of narcissist parents will either suppress their anger or turn it on themselves. When anger is internalized like this, people will criticize and find faults with themselves. They can end up extraordinarily depressed or even have suicidal thoughts; thoughts of suicide can be said to be the ultimate manifestation of anger in opposition to the self. Other people manifest their offense is in a passive-aggressive way, displaying behaviors like forgetting, lying, or avoiding. In this way, they are trying to get the better of their parents or person in authority.

They Interact with their Children by Emotional Contagion

Narcissist people, especially covert type, have minimal emotional experiences, and instead of talking about their personal needs, they usually act them out. The method of communication they use is known as emotional contagion. This communication method attempts to get other people to feel what they are feeling.

Emotional contagion is how babies and little children communicate. They cry until the people around them understand what is wrong and take steps to fix it. Emotional contagion from a distressed baby motivates a caretaker to do all they can to comfort the child.

Covert narcissist adults convey their feelings in this way. When they are distressed or upset, everyone around them scrambles to do all they can to make them feel better. In this way, the child catches the parent's distress and feels obligated to make the parent feel better. However, if the parent is unwilling to understand his/her feelings, nothing will ever get resolved. Instead, their upset feelings spread to everyone else so that everyone responds without truly understanding what the matter is.

They Avoid Doing Emotional Work

Narcissist parents never try to understand the emotions of other people. If they are accused of being insensitive, they dismiss the situation by claiming that the hurt person is overly sensitive. They attempt to rationalize their hasty and thoughtless responses. The way they respond shows that they cannot be bothered to take the effort to understand the emotions of other people, or are unable to

It Is Hard to Give Them
Narcissist parents want other people to pay attention to their needs, but it is tough to provide. They want others to show interest in their problems, but it is doubtful that they respond to helpful suggestions. They instinctively reject efforts to make them feel cared for. They drag other people in, but when they try to help, they chase them away. Instead of telling people what they need, they hold back, waiting to see if anyone will notice how they feel. They create a toxic guessing game that leaves everybody uneasy.

They Avoid Working to Repair Their Relationships
Problems will arise in a connection. When they do crop up, it is essential to work on addressing and solving the conflict. The skill to admit to being wrong and working on making things better requires maturity. Narcissist parents do not like to own up to their mistakes; they expect people to let them off the hook immediately. They can blame others if they are not forgiven immediately.

After a falling out, people try to repair the relationship by apologizing, seeking forgiveness, or making amends. This a repair attempt. Unfortunately, they utterly oblivious to what forgiveness means. Forgiveness to them means to make it as if the rift never occurred. They are completely unaware that people require emotional processing or time to rebuild trust after a falling out. The only thing they want is for things to go back to the way they were. The pain of others is unimportant.

They Expect Their Children to Mirror Them
Narcissist parents can reflect the feelings of their children by showing the same emotions on their faces. They display concern when their children are distressed and show enthusiasm when their children are delighted. In this manner, they teach their children about emotions and show them how to engage others spontaneously. It also gives their children the feeling of being seen and understood as a unique individual.

However, narcissist parents expect their children to understand and mirror them. They get extremely upset if their children do not act the way that they want them to. Unfortunately, it is not psychologically possible for a child to accurately mirror an adult.

They delude themselves into thinking that their kids will make them feel good about themselves. When their children start to develop their own needs, it can drive them to a state of intense anxiety. In some cases, they use threats of punishment and abandonment to gain control and reinforce their self-esteem at their children's expense.

Their Self-Esteem Is Dependent on Their Children's Compliance

For emotionally narcissistic people, they can only feel good about themselves when they can manipulate other people to give them their want and act the way they think they should. With their shaky self-worth, they find it difficult to tolerate the emotions of their children. If their child is upset, they start to question whether they are good or bad. If they cannot calm the child, they may feel like a failure and accuse the child of making them feel that way.

Their interactions with other people boil down to whether they are good people or bad ones. It clarifies their intense defensiveness if you attempt talking to them about something they did. They prefer to shut down communication, rather than listen to something that makes them feel like they are the wrong people.

Roles Are Sacred and Essential to Them

Role compliance is critical to narcissist parents. It helps to make life easy and allow decisions to be made more conveniently. They require their children to play a proper role, and that includes respect and obedience to them. They employ clichés to crop the dominance of their role as parents because they reduce the complexity of situations and generally make life easier. As a result of how essential roles are to them, they exhibit the following:

They Feel A Sense of Permission Because Of Their Social Role

It is a point of view that expects a specific treatment because of a social role. Narcissist parents behave as though being parents means they can stop respecting other people's boundaries or being considerate. When people feel entitled to act as they wish, this can be said to be role entitlement.

They Coerce Other People to Act Out Specific Roles

They can also compel other people to act out a role because they want them to. They force their children to act a certain way by not giving them the silent treatment, threatening to reject them, or getting other family members to attack them. When their children do things that they do not approve of, they make them feel guilty.

Narcissist parents are not comfortable with complex situations and prefer life simplified; thus, they have no hesitations about creating others' roles. If a person is not fulfilling a supposed role, something is wrong with them, and they need to change.

They Seek Enmeshment, Not Emotional Intimacy

Emotional intimacy and enmeshment are two ways of interaction that look similar but are very different. Emotional intimacy involves two individuals with a confident sense of self getting to deeply understand and know each other on every level and building emotional trust. This intimacy is refreshing and stimulates an individual's personal growth due to the interest and support that they enjoy from another person.

Each person plays a convenient role for the other, and by relying on this, they can flourish a sense of safety in the relationship. In cases where a person tries to detach himself/herself from the role, the other feels an apprehension that can only be eased by returning to the assigned role.

Their Poor Sense of Time Can Be Confused With Emotional Manipulation

It may look like emotionally immature people are emotional manipulators, but they are very cunning tacticians who press for whatever feels best at the time. They have no interest in being consistent; therefore, they say whatever grants them the upper hand at the moment, incredibly intense moments. In their work or other pursuits, they may think strategically, but they prefer to take an immediate advantage in emotional situations. An example of this is lying; it gives a quick-win that feels good at the moment, but it is detrimental to a relationship in the long run.

Narcissist parents see the family closeness and emotional intimacy as enmeshment. Real communication is almost impossible with them because of their low empathy and their insistence on roles. They neglect to repair their relationships and avoid the emotional work need to be thoughtful of other people, instead of focusing on whether other people make them look good or bad.

Chapter 8. Differences Between Male and Female Narcissists

Both male and female narcissists share their penchant for vying to be the center of attention, manipulating those around them, and superiority complexes. Still, there are some significant differences in preferred sources for their narcissistic supply and manipulation tactics they choose to employ between the genders. Generally, male narcissists are more overt, grandiose. They are typically diagnosed more frequently than women, whereas female narcissists are much sneakier and covert about manipulating and commonly classified as a vulnerable narcissist. By understanding the critical differences in how the different genders present themselves, you do not find yourself fooled by the less overt female narcissist who creates faux friendships to manipulate. Leaving those who do not understand narcissism thinks she cannot be a narcissist due to her being friendly with them. You will also understand the specifics behind the male and female's varying motivations, tendencies, and insecurities.

The Female Narcissist
The female narcissist is subtle in her narcissism; she prefers to go undetected, sucking up whatever attention she can get as needed. She likes to be the central focus and will use her appearance to her advantage. She often appears confident and comfortable in her skin and very embracing of her sexuality. She has no qualms over presenting herself as promiscuous and flirty to get what she wants. Because of this, she often

obsesses over her physical self, always appearing to be meticulously groomed and carefully selecting clothing, hairstyles, and makeup that allow her to present herself as conventionally attractive and higher class. Even those who were not blessed with perfectly symmetrical features appear entirely confident in their appearances. Which many people find beautiful, both romantically and platonically. Real confidence is attractive to other people as when someone is self-confident, they typically inspire confidence in themselves from those around them as well.

However, vanity has a downside, and female narcissists are much more likely to have an eating disorder than their male counterparts. It is due to female narcissists using their bodies as one of their manipulative tools. Their bodies must be perfect, and if they perceive themselves as too chubby, fat, lumpy, saggy, or flawed in any way, they fall into disordered eating to get their body to the proportions they deem as perfect. After all, narcissists expect nothing short of perfection.

Likewise, female narcissists take issue with aging, as the conventional beauty standard for women is achieved early to mid-20s. Once they have hit that peak, they become less and less conventionally attractive as they age. It is not meant to say that older women are less beautiful, but it highlights the female narcissist's obsession with self-image. She sees the hyper-sexualized ideal beauty in movies and media, and that is often younger women. Those features that make a woman conventionally attractive, symmetrical features, flawless skin, and a tight, fit body change over time. Like men, women begin to sag, wrinkle, and grey as the body ages, and the female narcissist sees this as the ultimate threat to her body's usefulness as a manipulative tool. It becomes something she is self-conscious of, desiring to be attractive because she believes her worth is in others' opinions of herself. She often thinks that being found appealing is the ultimate way of being desirable or valuable.

Unlike male narcissists, females are more inclined to seek their narcissistic supply at home from her family members, typically following conventional gender norms and seeing themselves as matriarchs to their families. It serves two purposes; it places them in a superiority position and likewise grants them control over their families. In preferring to use family to validate her ego, she uses her children as a primary source of her supply.

She will also tend to see her children as extensions of herself, and often project onto them. Her daughters will be more often seen as extensions of herself. In contrast, her sons will be put into a surrogate spousal position. The narcissistic mother will inappropriately confide in her son or put adult responsibility on him starting at a young age. She will groom him to fill the role a husband typically does, shaping him into exactly what she wants. She will take credit for any successes the children achieve, claiming that they could only score the winning goal because she gets up at 5 a.m. every morning to make them hearty, organic, homemade. Balanced breakfast, including using their chicken's fresh eggs and making the bread from scratch, get the nutrition they require. Those other kids who lost are malnourished and disadvantaged because their parents are nowhere near as good as her children.

Conversely, when her children fail or do something she disagrees with, she will make her displeasure clear, taking it as a personal insult. She may ask them why they did this to her and accuse them of intentionally doing it to hurt her. She will yell at and belittle the children that displease her, teaching them to walk on eggshells around them.

In romantic relationships, women often idealize and love bomb their target, seeking to make him or her intoxicated with her, so they want her around. She portrays herself as perfect, both in appearance and personality, and when he is hooked. She feels like he is no longer enough; she begins to emasculate him and break him down as a person until he is willing to accept her behavior and strive to please her. He may even tolerate her maintaining affairs with other men. One partner is rarely enough narcissistic supply, and she will seek as many sources of supply as possible, whether that is children, partners, or friends.

Females are also more covert in their rivalries with other women; they keep other women close and are very subtle about their criticism or belittling of others. Women's treatment often presents itself as a friendship if you are not well-versed in narcissistic tendencies and manipulation tactics. They seek to keep friends close, but only friends who are a little less pretty, a little less intelligent, a little less successful, or a little less wealthy than she is. None of her friends can better her in any way, or they will quickly find themselves discarded, as they no longer serve the purpose of making her feel better about herself and proving her as superior.

Female narcissists are much more materialistic than men and much more willing to spend frivolously. She doesn't feel the need to hoard her money to feel powerful; she loves to buy the newest, most excellent tech and fashion and flaunts it at every chance she gets. She thinks that spending money makes her powerful because others see her spending this money and assume she must be rich and influential. In reality, she is irresponsible and may even be accruing mountains of debt to maintain appearances. It allows the female narcissist to feel superior without being over-the-top about it; her accessories become her social status symbols. She never has to say a word about how great, consequential, or deserving she is; her appearance and actions speak it all.

The Male Narcissist

The male narcissist exhibits many more stereotypical traits of narcissism than the female; he is louder, more authoritative, and appears more overly confident than his female counterpart. He believes he is greater than the others and will assert this in any way he can, forcing others to submit to this belief. He often has much larger delusions of grandeur, in which he is the best simply because he is. Males care less about what other people think and are typically more likely to be grandiose narcissists. They seek power, control, and fulfilling their interests and let nothing stand in their way. Power and domination are essential for men, and they tend to gravitate toward more manipulative tactics and mind games as their tool of choice rather than sexual charm.

Male narcissists tend to cheat more often and are more likely to repeatedly cheat or carry on multiple affairs at one time, and seek gratification from their sexual relationships. Narcissistic men pursue numerous experiences to exert control and dominance; the more partners he has, the more dominant he must be, which is the opposite of the narcissistic woman, who seeks validation that she is attractive and desirable. He will feel powerful having multiple women at his disposal, and it is ultimately that power that he craves.

When it comes to children, men see them as an annoyance at best and competition for his narcissistic supply source at worse. Men typically use their wives or mothers as their primary sources of narcissistic supply. When children come along, naturally, the narcissist's wife will be spending ample time caring for the helpless newborn around the clock for at least a year and then spending the majority of waking hours catering to young children. Therefore, they naturally do not treat their children very well, and often assert as much control over their wives and raising the child as possible, perhaps saying he does not want to share. Therefore, she is not permitted to breastfeed or to insist that the child is left at his parents' home for long periods, so he has his wife to himself. Sometimes, he will project onto his children in a vulnerable narcissistic male and revel in the early affection and easy narcissistic supply earned from young children. Still, often, they reject their children as they grow up and become more independent.

In general, narcissistic men are less likely to spend money than their female counterparts, as to them, money is power, and they want to cling to as much energy as possible. That power grants them control over others and makes them feel important or as if they should be catered to. Especially in retail or customer service contexts, the narcissistic man will see his money as justification to treat the employee poorly. His money is enough justification that he is better than everyone else. Along with this, narcissistic men love to pursue high-paying jobs that grant them positions of power and control. If they cannot achieve these jobs, they aggrandize their positions. They are looking for any justification that they are superior to their coworkers and unreplaceable to their employment place.

Male narcissists see other men as their competition more so than a potential friend or ally. They are inclined to challenging other men, feeling threatened by their very presence, even if the other man is blissfully unaware of the threat he poses. He sees no reason to associate with other men unless it is to further his career or further dominate others. Rather than seeing any value in keeping male friendships, he treats other men as rivals superficially. He does not feel the need to seek validation from or justify his grandiosity with friends in the way the female narcissist does, as he is self-confident enough without it.

In this case, the narcissist either avoids performing or has a plausible, outside reason for his failure. Male narcissist is more likely than women to take part in this behavior, choosing behavioral handicaps such as alcohol or intentionally under preparing for something. In contrast, when women engage in this tactic, they prefer feigning illness or making up a trauma such as a friend or family member being injured or dying.

Chapter 9. Is a Hidden Narcissist Happy?

Despite how covert narcissists tend to present themselves, full of charisma and confidence, the inside is typically a broken, wounded individual with no real sense of self. They are not happy. The narcissist never had the chance to develop a normal, healthy. While some narcissists' lack of understanding of self is turned into a real, deeply held belief of superiority, many others are much more vulnerable. It is even a recognized kind of narcissism: Vulnerable narcissism. The narcissist feels inadequate and insecure and overcompensates with the boasting, tendency to manipulate, and creating a persona of the perfect victim that is never to blame for anything. These narcissists are overwhelmed with all sorts of secret feelings they aim to hide from public view at all costs, though their mask will fall under extreme stress or emotion.

Identity Crisis

Insecurity and vulnerability are at the foundation of many narcissists. Whether due to abuse during childhood or some other trauma, the narcissist has internalized that insecurity. Where most people have a voice that regulates their sense of self-worth, telling them that they are good enough and keeping them comfortable in their skin, the narcissist hears a voice telling her she is inadequate. Whatever she does is good enough for her, and she continually hears her inner voice putting her down. She always felt insecure in her skin and humiliated that she feels the way she does. The idea that the different people can see how insecure she is horrifying the narcissist because she thinks that admission of insecurity is an admission of weakness. The voices that shaped her poor sense of self-worth were correct. Other people acknowledging her insecurity makes her vulnerable, as that would be the easiest target to humiliate further and degrade her the first time she makes a mistake. Our parents or primary caregivers create that inner voice we all hear; the way our caregivers speak to us becomes the way we talk to ourselves. When our caregivers are overly critical, harsh, or cruel, their disapproval and loathing become internalized. We believe their word because, as children, we are hardwired to defer to our caregivers. We instinctively trust their judgments as correct because it is their job to help us learn to navigate through the world. The parent's role in a child's life is to teach the child how to be successful, well-adjusted, and all the skills they will need to cope with all of the turmoil that comes with being an adult. Sometimes, some parents fail miserably due to their abuse or lack the empathy and parental instincts required to be a successful parent. When parents continuously criticize or put down their children, their words become the child's frame for seeing the world around her.

When the child hears nothing but negativity and sees the world in that negative mindset, her entire way of thinking changes; she becomes insecure about everything, continually feeling incompetent and vulnerable. Her whole sense of self is shameful, negative, and self-loathing. With that loathing sense of self, she feels the need to overcompensate, and her behaviors become standoffish. She creates a persona focused on herself, pretending to be perfect, faultless, and likable to combat these feelings of worthlessness. By presenting as confident and perfect, and convincing others that this is who she is, she can protect herself from the harsh words she has come to expect from herself and others. She can sometimes convince herself that she is as confident and fantastic as she presents to those around her. However, she frequently swings right back to feeling insecure and vulnerable a short time eventually. Living in this nearly permanent state of insecurity leaves the narcissist continually feeling defensive and on edge, unable to relax for fear of someone around her taking advantage of her vulnerability and using it to climb the social hierarchy.

Issues with Intimacy

The intense levels of shame these narcissists feel act as deterrents from any real intimacy or relationships. Intimacy requires a vulnerability that the narcissist seeks to avoid at all costs, and therefore, it is avoided. The narcissist refuses to become vulnerable to others, seeking instead to protect her fragile ego from harm. She recognizes that being vulnerable means risking her ego being harmed, which is not a risk; she is willing to take. Vulnerability requires trust, and the narcissist will not trust anyone but herself. She knows that when she makes herself vulnerable, risks having the shame and self-loathing feel confirmed and validated by the person emotionally exposed herself to, and she refuses to risk that. Her fragile ego would not be able to take any criticism from someone she trusted, so instead, she decides to avoid trusting anyone at all.

Even though narcissists are emotionally stunted, they are typically quite intelligent and recognize a relationship between trust and vulnerability. Realizing that trust and openness are required for an intimate relationship, the narcissist instead decides not to commit. The relationship does not seem worthwhile enough, and the promise of intimacy is not enough for the narcissist to intentionally render herself vulnerable to someone else. Remember, her narcissistic behaviors are a coping mechanism to make herself invulnerable to harm; it would be counterproductive to go out of her way to become vulnerable, regardless of the reason. At the root of refusing to become susceptible is the shame and self-loathing that underlies all of her behaviors. She fears being humiliated, criticized, or harmed again, and that fear makes a connection with others quite difficult. Real intimacy is never achieved with the narcissist because of her narcissistic nature's existence as a coping mechanism. However, she will pretend and go through the motions of being in a relationship if she sees the benefit of doing so. It is important to remember, though, that she will never truly trust her partner and will never really make herself emotionally available or exposed.

Self-Direction and Deflection

While nobody enjoys being humiliated or embarrassed, narcissists fear humiliation more than anything else. Because narcissists already have impossible standards set for themselves and already see themselves as broken and fragile, having someone else makes them feel that way feels like salt in the wound. Knowing how weak they are and fearing that fragility being exposed, narcissists seek to avoid humiliation at all costs. Because the narcissist fears humiliation, she instead resorts to humiliating others around her. Rather than attempt to address any embarrassment on herself, she prefers to insult others, shifting negative attention away from her in ways that leave her blameless, but leave someone else being humiliated. It is another misguided coping mechanism; the narcissist feels too fragile, too self-conscious, and too vulnerable to survive humiliation, so she seeks to deflect it to others instead, even if they were just as undeserving and innocent as the narcissist. It also allows the narcissist to look better in comparison, providing an ego boost where there could have been ego injury.

The narcissist may point out a mistake someone else made, even if it was recently undetected. Even make up a mistake and blame it on someone else to keep potential negative attention away from her, even if there was little chance of negative attention being on her in the first place. Often, she fears humiliation from imagined sources, which is enough to send her on the defense. The most straightforward reason to make while maintaining an image of innocence is to force others to be defensive. After all, when everyone behaves defensively, no one is lashing out, and she remains unchallenged.

Undeserving of Empathy

One of the basic tenets of narcissism is the lack of or diminished capacity for feeling empathy. Lack of empathy makes it hard for the narcissist to imagine feeling deserving of compassion. Since empathy is almost foreign to the narcissist after a childhood of never having it emulated, she does not contemplate herself worthy of it. If she is not worthy, others must not be worthy either. It leaves her thinking the worst, rather than seeing that many humans are kindhearted and will go out of their way to help. Despite knowing the concept of empathy, it remains utterly foreign to her. Unless she is pretending for a good cause, it will never cross her mind to be empathetic with someone legitimately. Likewise, it would never cross her mind that anyone else would ever treat her with empathy. Even her parents, who were supposed to treat her with empathy and respect, never gave her that courtesy. She must be undeserving if even her parents could not manage to muster up enough care about her to treat her as a human with feelings that deserve to be recognized. Because of this belief of being unworthy of empathy or kindness, the narcissist views everything as suspicious. Nothing is to be trusted, and every action has an ulterior motive simply because the narcissist always has an ulterior reason. She refuses to see the best in others and cannot recognize that sometimes people do something out of their hearts' kindness to selflessly help others because the concept of selflessness is entirely foreign to her. Those behaviors were not modeled for her when they mattered, and she no longer considers them options.

This lack of deserving empathy paired with worthlessness creates even more feelings of inferiority, as the narcissist does not believe that making a mistake will be treated gracefully or kindly. She is confident that making a mistake is one of the worst-case scenarios and will reflect much worse on her than it actually will. Because of that, she will go to great lengths to hide any mistakes she may make, or push the blame away from herself, using any possible plausible deniability, no matter how realistic or ridiculous her excuse sounds.

Since she is unworthy of that kindness and believes that others will treat her poorly, it becomes easier for her to treat others unkindly instead of empathetically. It is a negative cycle of feeling others will treat her poorly because she is unworthy. Therefore, she will treat others that way preemptively to avoid being in a situation of vulnerability. She falls into this habit to protect herself and avoid exerting any energy she could use to better care for herself. Since others will not treat her with kindness or help her meet her needs without prompting, she feels driven to force the point and manipulate those around her to get what she feels like she needs or deserves.

Chapter 10. What are the Secret Methods in Which Hidden Narcissists use Social media

Technology always seems to have an upside and a downside. Computers and mobile devices certainly have improved communications and productivity. Social networking has been a great way to reconnect with old friends, meet people, and advance careers. But there could be a baited trap to this new online lifestyle, especially to young people, and it's not just possibly tripping into a fountain while walking and texting in the shopping mall. Many experts believe that the Internet and mobile computing may be breeding narcissists.

Early in life, everyone is narcissistic. But most people eventually learn to give up their juvenile self-centered attitudes and generally develop through social interactions with others. It is how most people know consideration, compassion, and empathy for others.

Narcissism and Social Networking

Did you hear about this book from a friend's post on your Facebook wall or via a tweet? If you did, that's a good thing. But a growing number of respected researchers are pointing to a possible link in the rise of narcissism in young people and the enormous popularity of social networking.

Social networking sites such as Facebook, Twitter, and YouTube are not all that "social" if you stop and think about it. In fact, in many ways, they are antisocial. Such sites allow you to socialize but are more like "mecentric" private clubs than any proper social environment. On a social networking site, you are entirely in charge of whom you will and will not interact with. You can quickly screen out those whose opinions differ from yours. Such sites are designed to build a network of growing fans and followers—a narcissist's dream!

No one says that if you or your kids or loved ones use Facebook, they will automatically turn into narcissists like in some bad horror movie. After all, there are more than 500 million users of Facebook at this writing, and not all of them are narcissists. But for a teen prone to the feeling she is a bit more entitled than others, who need to draw attention to herself, or who has a deep-rooted need to show the world just how great she is, Facebook is a great place to do so.

So, would you know if your loved one is using Facebook to feed narcissistic needs? Look for these signs:

Is she primarily using the site as a place to be "all about me"? Budding narcissists use Facebook for self-promoter, rather than to listen to and commiserate with their peers' problems and concerns. Look for the use of "me," "I," and "my" in every post.

Try to monitor how often she uses the site, maybe by seeing how many new Status Updates she makes every day. Does she feel she needs to check back often to see if her number of fans or friends has increased? Does she continuously feel the need to post such increases in connections as if it were a competition?

Watch for selecting her profile picture, and how often she feels the need to change it. Is it a simple snapshot, or does it always have to be the most glamorous picture, taken in an exotic locale? Is she wearing revealing clothes or dressed in a costume somehow?

If you ever see that a child under eighteen has posted sexual, violent, or inappropriate messages or pictures of herself online, you must act. If you are the parent, remove the images, delete the messages and the profile, and deny Internet privileges until your child learns the dangers of posting such things. If you are not the parent, notify the child's parents immediately. If necessary, inform the site's administrators, who will be more than happy to remove the inappropriate content from their network.

At its most basic level, narcissism is all about creating a falsified persona behind which the narcissist can hide her true feelings of self-loathing. There can be no better place to create a false identity, profile, or avatar than on the Internet.

Recognizing an Internet Narcissist

Social networking profiles and the like can tell you more than just people's birthdays, where they went to school, and their favorite movie; they can reveal many quirky personalities, including NPD.

Not everyone who asks you to be a friend on Facebook is a narcissist. Still, some telltale signs could reveal a narcissistic personality hiding behind an online facade. Just as in the real world, where narcissists surround themselves with many shallow relationships, those with vast numbers of online friends can be digital narcissists. Narcissists use online connections the same way they do every other relationship in their lives: to self-promoter, emphasizing quantity over quality.

Interestingly enough, since online narcissists tend to have infinitely more contacts than other users of such sites, you are far more likely to encounter narcissists within your group of online friends than you would in the real world. So, the more you use social networking sites, the more likely you are to become involved with a narcissist.

Narcissists are very susceptible to what clinicians have described as Internet addiction. On social networking sites, the narcissist can be the center of his world, attracting an ever-growing crowd of fans, friends, and followers. The digital narcissist can be treated to an almost unlimited source to feed his grandiose fantasies and inflated self-image, without any of the usual risks associated with his behaviors in the real world.

Narcissists, or people with narcissistic tendencies, can sometimes feel as if cyberspace, and in particular social networking sites, were created just for them. It is a world where false identities are not only acceptable but encouraged. The Internet world is bound by few rules or laws of societal norms—in other words, it's the perfect playground for narcissists.

If the bad news is that social media outlets on the Internet are crawling with narcissists, you can train yourself to spot them fairly quickly and promptly unfriend them. The problem is since you don't have a tone of voice, eye contact, or body language to go by, how do you spot a digital narcissist?

If someone's profile and the page give you the feeling that he looks as if he is a celebrity but not, it may be a good sign that he is a digital narcissist.

Not every profile you run into that shows these signs means you may be getting involved with a dangerous narcissist online. But just as you would in any potential relationship, use these signs as red flags and proceed with caution before answering that friend request!

Narcissism and Cyberbullying

If the Internet and social media sites are the ideal playgrounds for narcissists, you know every playground has its bullies. The recent, sometimes dangerous rise in cyberbullying is also related to the link between the Internet and narcissism.

Like any tool or technology, there are some excellent uses of the Internet. But the positive aspects of cyberspace are usually of very little interest to narcissists. The people in your life with NPD or narcissistic tendencies are not trolling around the Net looking to expand their horizons, develop new and positive relationships, or reconnect with old friends because they care about what is going on in their lives. If they could Google "narcissistic supply," they would, because that is the only thing they are searching for! They would get it in any means, including bullying and intimidation.

Avoiding the Trap of Internet Narcissism

So, if the Internet can be such an enabler of narcissistic tendencies, how can you or someone you know avoid being sucked into the trap of digital narcissism? The first thing you need to do is take a step back and regain a little perspective. It may be nice to let your online friends know what you are thinking, but just how important is it to broadcast what you feel every hour of every day? Try limiting your social-networking time to once or twice a week and then only to update people with really important or relevant information. Make it a competition with yourself: "Let me see if I can go without social media until Saturday!"

One of the best ways to avoid being led into digital narcissism is to prevent posting offensive, demeaning, or malicious statements by following the cardinal rule of If you wouldn't say it to a person, don't say it online. The Internet does not stop your words from hurting someone else. And worse, your comments can last forever online.

When you are online on any website, try limiting your visits to just a few minutes to catch a quick update or two. Don't spend hours and hours delving into other people's pages!

Try not to let your online identity dictate how you act, react, or participate in events in real life. For example, do not accept an invitation to a party so that you can put pictures of yourself being there on your online social-network "wall." Similarly, do not decline an invitation to a party you want to attend because you are afraid pictures of you might get posted on other people's online walls!

And finally, if you feel yourself being swept up into the temptation of digital narcissism, just quit doing social networking! Go cold turkey. You can cancel or temporarily deactivate your Facebook or Twitter account; many who have done so said it was the best decision they ever made.

Chapter 11. Exposing a Narcissist and Their Most Hidden Fears

It might seem like a good idea, in light of all you have just read. It isn't. If you threaten to expose the narcissist, then you will have a bloody war on your hands. Do not expect ever to put one over a narcissist, because it's not going to happen. The deviousness and cleverness of the narcissist are beyond anything you've ever encountered before.

Another reason you should not threaten to expose the narcissist is that while you might pull your punches as a decent human being, the narcissist has no depth; she will not sink to bring you down. He or She will not hold back, and nothing is off-limits. You cannot beat the narcissist at their own game, nor should you even bother trying. Their game is something they have played forever. They're comfortable with it. On the contrary, you do not have much experience as the narcissist, nor do you have the stomach for such vileness. It doesn't mean you should keep on being a victim. Just focus on yourself, not the narc. Focus on extricating yourself from their web and healing yourself from all the damage they have caused. If you're still hell-bent on showing the world that they are, then your best bet would be not to make a threat. Honestly, it's better to pack up and run than to stick around trying to prove yourself right. Sooner, the narcissist's dastardly deeds catch up to them. They will be exposed.

As confident and self-assured as the narcissist makes himself out to be, it's pretty intriguing that there are people the narcissist is deathly afraid of. If you could become this sort of person, you would find yourself less of a narc magnet. You'd be able to deal with all kinds of toxic people, or better yet, discard them before they're able to take a shot at you.

The Dissimilarity between the Narcissist and the Sociopath

The narcissist, unlike the sociopath, desires all the attention to be on them. They love to be admired. They love having their egos stroked. On the other hand, the sociopath does not give a rip what others think about her.

Since the narcissist craves the love, attention, and care of others, it becomes even more vital to keep their public persona intact. After all, who could love the real narcissist? Who could love someone so vile, cruel, and cold? They know that their authentic selves could never get away with even a teeny bit of the crap they do if the whole world gets to see them for what they are. It's because they know this that they fight tooth and nail to keep you, their source of attention and Achilles' heel, from ratting them out.

The narcissist is worried about being perceived as a cruel person. So, they make sure they have everyone who could buy into your story on their side. That way, even if they don't believe them over you, there is still room for them to doubt what you say about them.

What are the Most Hidden Fears of A Secret Narcissist?

- The narcissist is afraid of those who are more powerful than they are.
- They are scared of people who can harm them or undermine them in some way.
- They are afraid of people who will reveal them for what they indeed are.

But above anyone else, the person they fear the most is you. It might make no sense since if you're their victim, not the other way around. You are the person they fear the most because you, more than anyone else, know exactly who they are. You know the real monster behind their false persona. No one else does. Everyone thinks that they're the best person on earth, but you know better. It is why your abuser is scared of you. Because you're the only person who sees what the narcissist is, it means you alone can expose them. The narcissist cannot stand the thought of public humiliation, revealing their true, ugly glory. So, they do all they can to protect that facade. If you told someone about the things the narcissist does to hurt you, they would never believe you in a million years because of how carefully the narcissist has crafted their false image. It is also why the narcissist does all he can to discredit you at every turn and make you an outcast. Abuse from the narcissist comes from a place of fear-the fear of being unmasked once and for all.

You can't go around continuously rehashing everything the narcissist has done to you. It's no good for you, emotionally and physically. It's also not going to bode well for your future relationships. It is why you need to forgive the narcissist.

Forgiveness is not about letting them back into your life. It's helping you let go of all that angst and hurt, so you can move on with healing yourself. It is the only solution you can move forward. Forgiveness does not mean that you should start afresh with the narcissist, or keep letting them run you over. It means allowing yourself to move on.

It may seem easy to say, but one good thing to keep in mind to help you forgive the narcissist is that they do all they do because of a deep-rooted fear of you and all you stand for. Truthfully, a narcissist is a pathetic, sad sack of blood and bones masquerading as a human. There is no day the narcissist does not feel insecure and ashamed and guilty. The weight of all of that is too great for them to bear. So, they look to you, a paragon of all that they wish they could be but never will, as the perfect person to dump it all on, since they do not have the strength of character to face their inner demons.

These demons torment them, relentlessly, never taking a break. It is why the narcissist, in turn, relentlessly seeks others to torture, to rope into the anguish that she feels inside. That anguish is punishment enough. Let the knowledge of just how pathetic and helpless the narcissist makes it easier for you to forgive them, forget them, and move on with your life, a lot wiser and a lot stronger for it all.

Narcissistic Projection

Because the narcissist is deathly afraid of the potential power you have to bring him or her down, they will embark on the biggest, most extensive smear campaign they can, so that you lose all integrity in the eyes of those who would have listened to you.

You'll notice a fascinating thing about the narcissist's smear campaign: It involves projection, lots and lots of it. What this means is that the narcissist will accuse you of everything that they have done to you. They're the ones who are guilty of these crimes but never mind that. They can pin it on you. They do precisely that.

The narcissist will always project all the stuff they're guilty of. They cannot help themselves. A surefire way for you to figure out all the heinous things the narcissist has been up to is to pay attention to the things they accuse you of. If they charge you of cheating, stealing, or whatever, other unimaginable things that tumble out of their mouth, then we bet you dollars to donuts that they have done all that, and then some.

Say the narcissist you're dealing with happens to be a colleague at work. The narcissist will go around telling others that you're sabotaging him. He'll spin tales about how you deliberately make the office uncomfortable for him. He'll tell people about how you're always telling a lie after lie about him to anyone willing to listen. See the irony in this? The narcissist is doing precisely what he's accusing you of!

When the Narc Calls You a Narc

Remember, the narcissist is only projecting. They're super smart. What another way to not be seen as a narc than to accuse you of being one? You're the problem. You're the one always causing all the issues at work or in your relationship.

The narcissist will rope others into making them believe you're the one who's the rotten egg, and they should cut you off. When this happens in your workplace, it can have very dire consequences. You might find yourself out of a job because everyone is singing the songs about you that the narc has taught them to upper management. More often than not, victims of workplace narcissists end up leaving their jobs or getting fired. The sad thing is that the truth can take a long time before it finally is revealed. The narcissist is always searching for a target and collecting them. Eventually, the people in your life — whether they be your bosses or your loved ones who the narc has cut off from you — will come to realize what happened.

Chapter 12. A Hidden Narcissist Suffers Internally?

Narcissists are continuously overlooked to be good characters. Yet they are vulnerable people who need an understanding of oneself. They create their model and standing throughout others and require self-identity when isolated.

They are usually scared of getting a proper study of themselves because the consequences would be frightening. Many of them are spiritually wasted, so they must explore support from another person. When neglected to study about a narcissist, you will describe an egotistic character who has an overblown personality. In reality, they cannot live in a lack of their martyrs because they depend on others to utilize their thinking and attitudes.

Their thinking is defined by anxiety, uncertainty, and delusions. The unenthusiastic character controlled by most of them serves to give them weak, helpless, and hurt. They continue visualizing themselves as higher, yet when it is evident, this is impossible.

Narcissistic behaviors are often based on certain mindsets and beliefs that associate power with another people's ill-treatment. This belief system makes narcissists view their peers as weak and inferior people who do not need any attention. A narcissist person also believes that a person's worth is derived from his superiority or inferiority level. These attributes are exhibited through certain emotions like rage and anger. The mentality of a narcissist can cause him to detach from the feelings of others. It explains why most narcissists will never connect with the pain and challenges of their peers or relations. It also explains why they will always dismiss complaints arising about them.

In the mind of a narcissist, the partnership does not need to exist in relationships. To him, any relationship must have a top dog and an underdog. The narcissist will continuously fight to be superior or the top dog. The general belief is that human beings can either rule or be ruled. Such a mentality causes narcissists to feel entitled to a certain kind of treatment.

Another mindset assumed by narcissists is that people are only there to serve their needs. That's why they ignore others' needs because they think others do not need comfort and assistance. To them, it is the responsibility of their partners to serve and provide comfort. The narcissist wants to be adored, praised and valued all the time.

In a nutshell, live with a narcissist is all about competition. Narcissists will compete with their colleagues, family members, and partners to ensure that they remain in control. Due to this, narcissists never rest. To ensure They stay on the offensive side to keep others admiring their courage. Their behavior revolves around building their status and building their interests.

Here is the thought pattern of a narcissist who is always wired differently. Let us look at some of the common thoughts that keep running through their mind:

- 'Why am I not getting the attention I need?'
- 'I only need to concentrate on myself and take care of my own needs.'
- 'I need to get out of this relationship because I do not feel in control.'
- 'I am always right, you are always wrong, and you can do nothing about this fact.'
- 'Why do I need to feel bad for someone else?'
- 'I deserve some appreciation, why have I not received it?'
- 'I feel bored; it's time to stir things up.'
- 'Why do you think you are to cause me shame?'

Narcissists will avoid every activity or behavior that can make their codependents feel appreciated. Their strategies are fashioned towards tearing others down. For a narcissist, there is the only method of winning – controlling the mind of other people. Sadly, with all the attention and admiration they receive, they rarely get pleased. They can only feel suitable for a short while, then get back to doing hurtful things to remain in dominance. That is why most of them stay miserable for a good part of their life.

Chapter 13. Benign and Malignant Narcissism (Overt and Covert)

People whose focus is always on their own needs are narcissists; they find it very difficult or impossible to consider others' feelings. They do not possess any understanding of compromise, respect, or integrity. The only care about their desires and make an enemy of anyone or anything blocked them from getting it. Remorselessness, selfishness, shallowness, and sadistic nature are a real narcissist feature, and they can be of any gender, age, race, or sexuality.

What is a Benign/Covert Narcissist?

The benign narcissist has had a tough life, terrible relationships, and challenging childhood; thus, he is a professional victim because he has experienced several tragedies. The benign narcissist has never experienced love, everyone in his life has left him, and most of his attempts have proven abortive. He is obsessively attached to his partner, recognizing him as a narcissist difficult, which is dangerous. You can only start to find out how selfish they are after you have known them for a while. We confuse selfishness with insecurity as he always puts his needs first.

Empaths are mainly attracted to a benign narcissist; this is because he makes his neediness obvious, and people like empaths who want to help him get attracted. The benign narcissist is more like a predator that tricks his prey by pretending to be injured. It also seems to be worse than the overt narcissist because the overt narcissist makes victims conform to the idea that they need him to survive. In contrast, the covert narcissist inculcates the impression he requires so much of the victim's help. The malignant narcissist uses fear and abuse to checkmate his victim, whereas the covert narcissist employs sympathy. Since the covert narcissists portray themselves as needy, it is difficult for their victims to leave.

What is a Malignant/Overt Narcissist?

Our initial thought when we are thinking of narcissists is that of an arrogant blowhard with no belief of ever being wrong, or that they are a gift of God to humans, they are the malignant or overt narcissists. This type of narcissist is over narcissistic, the word means not hidden or seen, and this is a clear definition of an overt narcissist. It is an egotistical, arrogant narcissist who is not a bit scared of tooting his own horn. Instead, he is proud of it and expects the same from every other person; he tends to be sadistic, condescending, cruel, cold, and sarcastic. His character is not sympathetic; he gets appalled when challenged and insists that his desires will be catered for instantly. Every piece of individuality in their partner will be destroyed; his thinking will replace it. He seldom bullies, cheats and physically abuses the partner. He believes in entitlement to all his wants and makes unfathomable entitlement statements while keeping a straight face. Though he sometimes is smooth and looks like someone who has everything together, he is shockingly selfish and scary.

It is a prominent type of narcissist but very dangerous; therefore, their personality cannot be mistaken. They shove everything they do on your face. The malignant narcissists possess an easily-crumbling perfected smooth facade, which helps them attract friends and partners. It easily crumbles because of their vast poisonous ego, which commands acknowledgment. Due to this, they seem easily avoided compared to their counterpart, the covert narcissists

The Difference

The benign narcissism and malignant narcissism do not have much difference. The benign narcissist makes plans to make sure that they meet his needs differ from that of the deadly, though there is no much difference in their markets. Instead of a malignant narcissist to attack, physically abuse, or blackmail with murder, which the benign narcissist will employ, they will instead use sympathy or suicide attempt, but they are all the same. For this example, both of them have the same insinuation.

There are rare cases where the two types of narcissists employ abuse, and also there are scenarios where they both use sympathy, which is because the overt and the overt are only facades. You can get rid of the front for the screaming, wounded child concealed to be exposed, and this is similar for both types of narcissists.

Their choice of self-presentation for both types of narcissists has a reference to the original personality before them receiving the narcissism wound, which has reformed them into their current self and gives the much manipulation advantage. The malignant narcissist has earlier inculcated the bullying mentality, perhaps because it has a connection to the personality. In contrast, the covert narcissist has conformed to the belief that employing sympathy and guilt will better work for him.

It could also be affected by the narcissist's personality disorder. They can further deduce that benign narcissism has a borderline disorder, while the malignant personality is associated with a psychopath. There might be a complication when considering a cluster B personality disorder victim who tends to have more than one disorder type, which results in the display of several behaviors.

In a scenario where one person manifests narcissistic, borderline, and antisocial personality disorders, several signs of a covert narcissist will be portrayed and an overt narcissist. This person tends to cry and appear sympathetic when appalled, although he still has a feeling of being humiliated, or he may display violence and threats. This behavior tends not to blend with that of a sympathetic action (i.e., I am needy, I am a toxic waste, I am helpless, and I am a victim). The occurrence is inevitable because every type of narcissism possesses a massive core that involves a defective, poisonous, and colossal ego. This stated ego requests punishment when it is acknowledged.

Chapter 14. How your Life Changed when you Left a Narcissist

After the storm, when the waves of the emotional seas calm down a little bit, and you can feel a new attitude and outlook on your life journey, you may still have a lot to do to help yourself recover from your awakened awareness of your situation. If you have chosen to stay in your relationship with your partner because you want to heal yourself from within that dynamic, then some of this guide will not help you.

When you are in a narcissistic abuse situation, the best recourse is to remove yourself from gaining insight. Surviving a narcissistic relationship and staying with a partner who has this personality disorder can be a very one-sided battle that you will fight alone. You will have to decide what is essential for you over your relationship with yourself.

Breaking away from the narcissistic abuse cycle patterns is best achieved by letting go and moving on. Even if you have ties that keep you together, like children, or other matters, you can still succeed and thrive after the storm has calmed, and you have moved forward and onward. To fully heal from the cycles of abuse, the toxic patterns of narcissistic partnership, and the emotional manipulation you endured, you will have to do much personal growth work to support your choice. Remove any doubts that you have made the right choice. Being mentally manipulated for a period is not without its damaging side effects, and it could take some time for you to end the emotional upheaval you experienced.

The person you were involved with may still try to convince you that you have something unique and make a huge mistake. Or you may find yourself head over heels with another partner soon after you end your relationship, who also happens to be a narcissist. However, you couldn't see the red flags because of how close you still are to those behaviors, thoughts, and emotional patterns.

It will serve as an inspiration for you to heal the patterns of narcissistic abuse and relationships so that you can seek out a healthier relationship with yourself and someone else in your future.

After You Walk Away

After you walk away from a narcissistic partnership, you may go through several feelings of doubt, uncertainty, "but what if's" and all sorts of highs and lows that will want you to question if ever you have made the right choice. You will always have to work out your version of what happened in your relationship with your partner, and they are not going to be willing or able to face the trauma you experienced. Your narcissistic partner won't even care that you are or were in pain, or that you felt emotionally abused. Anything that comes up and suggests that you are doing something wrong, or making the wrong choice by leaving your partner, is just more of the toxic reality of being a victim of narcissistic abuse rearing its head.

The following methods will help you stay focused on getting through the hard parts of walking away and how to continue healing the patterns of the narcissistic relationship and cycles of abuse.

Process Your Emotions

Spending time with your feelings, honoring them, labeling them, and acknowledging your experiences and the events of your relationship will help you manage the reality of what you experienced more efficiently and effectively. When you can explore what happened from a distance, you will have a clearer perspective instead of from the relationship's confines. You can even try to imagine how it would look if it happened to someone else, like a friend or a colleague, to help you see more objectively and process your feelings from various angles.

Using a journal or notebook, seeking counseling, and asking for support in a group can also help you process your emotions more effectively. You don't have floods of feelings or doubts about your process as you change course and create a new life for yourself.

Keep It Personal, and Try Not to Generalize
It would be effortless to become cynical and embittered about anyone in the world after an experience of narcissistic abuse. Creating a shield of armor to prevent further issues can be even more damaging. The tendency might be to generalize the situation to say, "All women are control freaks," or "all men are manipulative masochists," but that is not the case or the answer to your healing dialogue. Take time to reflect as a unique experience and not the assumption of all society, men, women, or anything.

A Little Self-Compassion Goes A Long Way
You might not be practiced anymore at offering yourself compassion. How could you be after living with a narcissist who is the antithesis of compassion and empathy? Pitying yourself or being overly critical of your experience will keep you locked in patterns of self-abuse, the learned behavior of emotional manipulation you gained in your relationship. The antidote to those feelings is self-compassion, which could take some practice at first, little by little, and add up over time, supporting you in a much healthier way.

Be fair, and do not judge yourself too much. Be understanding that you are not a fool for getting involved with someone like that; they are incredibly charming and warm when you first get to know them and incredibly skilled at convincing you of anything. You are not stupid. So, be kind and understanding in the face of the narcissistic aftermath. Recognize that thousands of people find themselves in these circumstances and that you are one of many people who were a victim of narcissistic abuse. We all have lessons to learn, and we are all working with the people and ourselves in our lives to figure it all out.

The High Road Is the Road to Take
Reacting to your narcissistic ex is not always easy to avoid, incredibly when provoking you and looking for a confrontation to prove a point.

Take the high road in every situation. It may feel awkward and uncomfortable at the moment because you have to put with their antics. Still, you will find a sense of relief, calm, and responsibility for your emotional agility when you choose the path that reflects a more grounded, resourceful, and wise individual.

Everything in recovery and moving forward is a stepping-stone. It may feel like a long haul, but every choice you make every day to help yourself let go and move forward healthily is what takes you to the path you truly want to be on as you create a happier and more fulfilling life for yourself.

Know the Flags

The best path to put yourself out of narcissistic coupling and abuse patterns is to make sure you know and understand all of the flags. Understanding what narcissism is and how it can manifest is an important thing to study.

If you are recovering from this type of relationship, you will be much more likely to spot a flag from a mile away. However, even still, narcissists can be incredibly cunning and slippery and are willing to do whatever it takes to convince you they are 100 percent compatible with you.

Researching your own experience and finding out all of the specific experiences as you process, journal, and speak to a therapist, will help you prevent a future narcissistic relationship. Watch out for the following flags as you meet new people and embrace contemporary romances:

- Idolizing you in front of friends and family to an extreme degree
- Love-bombing
- Whirl-wind getaways in a concise period
- Promising things and not sticking to those promises
- Having manic episodes of radical love expressions
- Excessive sexual needs
- The subtle devaluing of your efforts or feelings
- Not taking the blame for anything
- Never apologizing
- Expecting your love without offering much in return

This list is just the beginning before things get worse, and you don't want them to get worse, so heading it off at the pass with these first few red flags is a good plan. Some healthy and stable relationships start with a powerful and romantic bang; however, some excessive love demands can lead you toward knowing that you are dealing with a narcissist. This guide is your answer to making sure you understand how that looks.

Seek Help

You are not alone, and many people have experienced or experienced what you are going through. Ask for help, don't be afraid, and find a support system to offer you what you need to stay balanced, secure, and self-confident in your choices and journey forward.

It has never been your fault that the person you are in a relationship with doesn't understand their disorder or issue. Even if you were capable of enabling it for an extended period, you are certainly capable of healing from it and learning how not to repeat the same patterns repeatedly.

Help is always available and all around you. If you cannot get to a public support group, or feel comfortable talking to friends and family about it, go online and look for more resources. Find an anonymous group to join if you want to protect your identity. Ask other people about their experience and how their recovery process is going. You will learn so much by merely reaching out for help and letting it clear your fears that you are somehow at fault for your experience.

As you move forward, use this guide to help refresh your decision to move on. All it takes is awareness and courage as you let go of the narcissistic relationship. Empowering yourself to enjoy your Life more through a balanced partnership is what any person deserves, and you are on the correct road to getting there. Heal the patterns so that it cannot be repeated by offering yourself kindness. Staying personal with your journey, process your emotions regularly, take the high road, know the narcissist's red flags, and seek help whenever you feel like you need support.

You are on your way to becoming the confident, happy, and balanced person you always knew you could be and are. Learning to survive the narcissistic relationship may seem hard at first, but you have all of the tools you need to accept your story and begin the healing journey.

Chapter 15. Dangerous Covert Narcissist & Their Betrayals

Psychologists have stated what we are experiencing an epidemic of narcissism. They are dangerous, and they will betray you in every means! These toxic people are everywhere, and the chances are that you will cross paths with one in your life. They exist in our social circles, at work, in our schools, and our families.

While a narcissist may seem wise and cunning, the truth is that it is effortless for us to predict their behavior. Simply knowing what you should look out for will allow you to understand if a narcissist is manipulating you.

It may be true that we are experiencing an epidemic of narcissism, and here are the danger signs that you would like to take down to avoid their betrayals:

Always the Victim

The narcissist is still going to play the victim. While it is true that everyone can be a victim in some way, the narcissist will always portray themselves as the victim. The narcissist is going to believe that they are the victim in every circumstance. They will think that everyone is trying to take advantage of them, tell you that everyone is mean to them, and they are going to cry louder than those who are actual victims. The cause for this is that they know people are compassionate. They will use this compassion to show them to lure them in and get the attention they desire.

Is there someone you know that always seems to be the victim? Do they continuously tell you stories about how a person did something to them, and they don't even know why? Does it seem like details are being left out of their story? Are you wondering why so many people would victimize this one person?

If this is the case, it is likely that this person is a narcissist and uses these stories to get you to feel sorry for them.

Diversion Techniques

It usually happens when you have called the narcissist out on their behavior or caught them in a lie. They will throw statements at you such as, "I guess you have never told a lie," or "Oh my god, I made a mistake, sorry we can't all be as perfect as you."

It is a diversion. The goal is to catch you off guard, take the focus off of them and on to you, and cause you to sympathize with them. Of course, you know you are not perfect, and you know what it feels like to make a mistake. You know that everyone has told a lie at some point.

When the narcissist brings the attention off of them and onto you, they would make you think and feel that you were in their position. Then they can bend your will to what they want. They have an explanation for their behavior, and they know that it is one that you are willing to accept.

Sudden Changes in Behavior

When a person first meets a covert narcissist, they are made to feel as if the narcissists' world revolves entirely around them. They are flooded with praise and compliments, which creates a sense of security, even though it is false. The covert narcissist's goal is to cause you to become dependent upon the praise that they are showering you with. That's when things start to change.

Suddenly you are no longer receiving all of those compliments. You are not as wonderful as they once thought you were. Instead, they are calling you all sorts of names, belittling you, and beating you down emotionally. Their goal is to make you beg for the praise they used to provide for you; they can make you do whatever they ask.

Going on A Guilt Trip

Most of the time, when a covert narcissist uses guilt trips, they are a parent or other member of the family. They will begin by trying to make the victim feel guilty for something, and then they will tend to ask for something. For example, "Your brother came for a visit today. Why didn't you visit? Oh, I need you to bring me some money, you can visit then."

The guilt trips are used to make you feel like no matter what you have going on or how over-extended you already are, you need to find time to make up for what you have done wrong. The narcissist is not going to try to see things from your point of view.

"I was busy working all day, the kids still haven't had dinner, and I have a report due in the morning."

"But I am your mother, and this is the least you could do for me."

They do not care that you are doing all that you can, that you are exhausted, stressed, and that your plate is full. All they see is the chance to take advantage of your guilt and get what they want.

Aggression

When most of us think of aggression, we think of something that would push us away from a person; however, when a covert narcissist uses aggression toward their victims, it is meant to pull them in closer. As strange as it may seem, men and women alike have an attraction towards aggression. Women are usually more attracted to aggression than men, but men find themselves in this situation.

The reason that humans are attracted to aggression is primal. It is based on natural selection. When we have an aggressive partner, we are safe from those who would try to do us harm. The narcissist will feed off of this instinct. They know that if you do not do what they say or want, they can use their aggression to trigger this instinct. They will become aggressive, you will become more attracted to them without having any control over it, you will give them what they want, and they will maintain power over you.

Hoarding Conversations

All narcissists love to talk about themselves. They don't want to hear about you, your feelings, or your views. If you can get a word in on the conversation and it does not agree with what the narcissist is saying, they comment most likely to be dismissed, corrected, or ignored. The covert narcissist will want to make sure that they show you that they know more than you. They may respond to your comments with, "well, actually…" or "but…" to prove that they are superior.

They will try to ensure that the conversation is focused on them and what they think, but they will interrupt conversations that they are not a part of.

Breaking Rules

Narcissists are known as rule-breakers. They enjoy getting away with breaking the rules like stealing, jumping in line ahead of those that have been waiting, and even breaking laws. They feel that they are the exception to the rule. The rules do not apply to the narcissist as far as they are concerned, and if they want to break the rules, they have a free pass to do so.

They believe that the rules only suitable for us, ordinary people. The narcissist believes that if it were not for the rules, we would have no idea how to survive, but since they are so smart and so much more important than the rest of us, the restrictions do not apply.

Projecting a False Image

A covert narcissist wants to impress people by the way that they look on the outside. They hide their inside personality because it is so ugly that we would all run the other direction if we saw it.

The narcissist sees themselves as a trophy, and they want other people to see themselves as one as well. This complex can show its face in many different areas of the narcissist's life, including professionally, sexually, financially, socially, physically, and so on.

They want people to believe that they are the best at everything because this helps relieve the inadequacy that the narcissist feels about who they are. If they can persuade everyone else that they are as wonderful as they want them to believe, no one will ever know that they are inadequate. The difference is that the narcissist does not focus on accomplishments because they want to fulfill their goals; they only focus on them because they know it will get them their attention.

Entitlement
We have heard this word thrown around so much over the past few years. It seems that if someone wants to insult someone else, they call them entitled. In truth, entitlement means that a person has a right to something.

The narcissist believes that they are unique, more special than any other person put on this planet. They think that they should get whatever they want simply because they exist.

You will also notice that they have double standards. For example, you can never be late or take time to relax, but they can. You cannot talk to them a certain way, but they can speak to you that way. They are unable to compromise. They prioritize, and they believe that their needs should always come first even if it hurts other people.

As you can see, a person who has a sense of entitlement has a lot in common with a narcissist. The two problems overlap a lot of the time.

Charming
Narcissists tend to be very lovely. They are charismatic and very persuasive. They are great at making a person feel special and wanted when they first meet them before the abuse begins. However, once they have gotten what they want from you when they lose interest or have gained control over you, they have no problem dropping you.

The problem comes when the victim finds out who the person is. The victim will be tortured at the narcissist; however, most people will not believe what the victim says about the narcissist because that is not the person they see. Instead, they see exactly what the narcissist wants them to see.

Grandiose
The covert narcissist may think of themselves as heroes, or a princess, or just an extraordinary person. Their feeling of self-importance is exceptionally exaggerated. They believe that other people are not going to be able to survive without them. They think that somehow their contributions are magnificent.

They may even voice this opinion, "I don't know how you guys would survive if it were not for me." "I know when I am gone, this entire family is going to fall apart." "I saved the day; without me, you all wouldn't make it."

Negativity

The narcissist enjoys making people feel negative about themselves, their lives, the situation that they are in, the people around them, and everything else in their lives. They enjoy spreading the negativity around. It allows them to be the focus of attention and to feel powerful. It ensures that their victims remain insecure as well.

If you feel that a covert narcissist is manipulating you, you must start acting right now, distance yourself, and the narcissist. At this very beginning, your main goal should be to stop the manipulation and their betrayals to take control of your own life.

Chapter 16. The Most Common Phrases of A Secret Narcissist

If you have ever been in a relationship with a narcissist - or any toxic person for that matter - you understand how they use language to manipulate you. They use specific phrases daily to be used in a completely different text if they were not narcissists.

Studies have shown that a narcissist enjoys manipulating kindhearted people; they view it as a kind of sport. They believe that they are superior. By using you, they are building on this belief even when all of the evidence points otherwise.

They will use conversations as a way to bring you down or terrorize you. They will cause you to be so afraid to disagree with what they say that you will give up and agree with them. To understand what a narcissist means when talking to us, we have to decode their language. These phrases below are the most commonly used by narcissists, followed by what the narcissist means:

"I love you." – I love being able to control you, use you, and own you. I love that I can sweet-talk you, make you believe that I care about you, and toss you to the side as I please. I love that I can get whatever it is that I want when I flatter you. I love that you have opened up to me even though you were mistreated in the past. I love knowing that I can pull the rug out from under you whenever I want, and watch you crumble.

"I'm sorry."– I am not sorry. I want this conversation to end so that I can continue enjoying taking advantage of you. I do not care that you were hurt by what I did. I am only sorry that I was caught. I do not like that you are calling me out and holding me accountable for my actions. I wouldn't say I like dealing with your emotions. They are not valid as far as I am concerned because they interfere with me getting what I want. I do not care how you feel.

"You are overreacting" or "too sensitive." – While you may be having a perfectly normal reaction to all of the abuse that I have put you through, I do not like that you are starting to recognize what is going on. I am going to gaslight you to ensure that you continue to second-guess yourself. I know that you will continue to deny the abuse that I am putting you through if you do not trust yourself. You will rationalize my behavior, blaming yourself for it. While you are busy blaming yourself, you will be working very hard to keep me happy. I get all of the benefits without any of the consequences.

"You are going crazy." – I know that you are not crazy, but I love provoking you and making you think you are losing your mind. By pointing my finger and saying that you are the crazy one, I can make sure that the focus is taken off of me and put back onto you. It doesn't matter anyway. I have ensured that no one is going to believe anything that you have to say. They already know how unstable you are. I can make them feel anything about you.

"My ex is crazy." – My ex is not crazy, and if he/she is fantastic, it is because I made them that way. I had so much fun, torturing, provoking, and agitating them. I was always able to get a reaction out of them, which I used to prove to everyone how crazy they were. Don't worry; I'll tell everyone how crazy you are as well.

"They are just a friend." – I keep him or her around in case you start to bore me. If I ever get tired of you or begin to bore me, they could be your replacement. They are already taking your place when I don't feel like being around you. If you complain about what I am doing, I am going to make sure that everyone believes that you're the one who is trying to control me. I will make sure that you seem like the abusive one.

"Stop being so jealous." – I love making you jealous. I love that you are willing to compete with other people for my attention. It makes me feel so powerful, knowing that I can make you jealous so easily. I can create insecurities within you merely by flirting with another person. The more insecure you feel, the more powerful I think. Everything that you believe is going on is, but there is nothing that you can do about it. I am qualified to do whatever I want with whoever I want.

"Your trust issues are not my fault." – Sure, I know that you should not trust me. I know that I will go behind your back whenever I want and do whatever I want, but I'm not going to admit that to you. It would probably be best if you trusted your instincts and got away from me as quickly as possible, but then I wouldn't be having any fun. I enjoy seeing you question your instincts.

"It's not always about you." – It's never about you. It is always about me. If you ever decide to start focusing on what you want or need, I will make sure that you feel like the most self-centered person on the planet. I will make sure that you feel guilty for even considering taking care of your own needs. I have no desire to fulfill your needs; I couldn't do it if I wanted to. But I don't want to.

" Can we still be friends?" – I hate to see someone that I worked so hard to train disappear. I like keeping track of all of my exes. That way, whenever I need some extra reassurance, they are right there for me to start manipulating all over again. Staying friends makes it easier for me to keep a hold on you. This way, you will never indeed be free of me.

"No one will ever believe you." – I have made sure that you are completely isolated and have no one to turn to for support. I have destroyed your reputation, ensuring that everyone believes every lie that I have ever told about the person you are. If you go looking for help, not one person will believe what you tell them, and they are all still going to think that I am unique.

"You're never going to find another person like me." – It will probably be a perfect thing if you never find another person like me. If you discover your worth, you could leave, and then I have to start all over with another victim. I would instead you continue trying to make me happy.

Knowing the most common phrases that narcissists use and what they mean is only half of the battle; it is also essential for you to understand how to react to what the narcissist is saying. When you know ahead of time how you will respond to what the narcissist in your life says, you will remain calm and in control. It will infuriate them because they will begin to see that they do not have control over you any longer. They will recognize that you are starting to take control back from them.

One of the biggest mistakes people make when they come face to face with a narcissist is trying to get the narcissist to see the logic. You cannot use sense when a narcissist wants to start an argument.

You will need a few strategies of your own that will help you stay grounded when the narcissist tries to attack you verbally. These strategies allow you to control your emotions, even when the narcissist is trying to make you lose control. These five statements can be used whenever you feel that the narcissist is trying to take power from you.

"Thank you for informing me how you feel." You can use this phrase whenever you have a conversation with a narcissist, and they are trying to blame-shift. It shows them that you will not allow it to affect you emotionally while you have heard what they have said. After you have made this statement, you will go back to focusing on whatever your point was before they started trying to blame you for the situation.

"I wanted you to know how I feel." We are all tempted to try and ensure that the narcissist knows how we feel; we hope that if they start to understand how they make us think, they will change their behavior. But they are not going to know how you feel, nor are they going to care. They know that you want them to understand the damage they are doing, but they will ensure you only get the opposite of what you are asking as a narcissist. We all need to be able to express ourselves and our feelings. Saying, "I wanted you to know how I feel" allows you to express yourself while maintaining emotional control. Once you have made this statement, you will end the conversation right there.

"Thank you for expressing your opinion." You can use this phrase when the narcissist goes on and on about a specific thing or evidence that they are just trying to get a reaction out of you. Using this phrase allows the narcissist to express their "feelings" as we all should be able to do, but it also shows them that you will not lose control of your emotions no matter what their opinions are. When you use this phrase, you do not tell them that you agree with their statement or tell them that your idea is wrong. Instead, you ensure that you do not feel the desire to have the same views as the narcissist. You will never have the same opinions as them, no matter how much they try to force you to do so.

"I'm sorry that you feel like that." You can use this when the narcissist starts using name-calling or tries putting you down.

Using these phrases allows you to remain calm and think more clearly. When you allow a narcissist to upset you emotionally, you cannot think clearly about the situation. The narcissist is counting on this happening because they know that if they can keep you from thinking clearly, they will maintain control over you.

While nothing will stop the narcissist's behavior, using the techniques you have learned in this guide will allow you to block their action from affecting you. What is essential is that they will see that you will not allow them to victimize you, and while that will drive them crazy, they will usually become bored and go looking for a new victim.

Chapter 17. Is A Narcissist Intelligent?

Narcissists are often intelligent people who use gaslighting to control their victims' thoughts and emotions. Gaslighting is a form of psychological manipulation used by the narcissist to make victims count on them for world perceptions.

Gaslighting is done in the subtlest of ways, and so the signs are easy to miss. The way gaslighting is carried out is why smart people can easily fall victim to this favorite narcissist weapon.

So why does gaslighting work so well on intelligent people?

Well, gaslighting works on the most intelligent people for several reasons:

- Smart people often possess the tendency to project their morality, empathy, and conscience onto others.
- Most intelligent people tend to project their qualities of empathy and good conscience onto others. They believe other people will act with the highest moral standards too.
- They are emphatic people who feel other peoples' feelings strongly. They walk into the room and immediately spread good energy, and so their genuine feelings for others often lead them to the error of believing that everyone has real feelings for others.
- Intelligent people will assume the best about everyone, and this belief will mean they do not readily see that they are being manipulated.

- Narcissists naturally gravitate to those who have the qualities they admire.
- Too often, intelligent people attract narcissists not only because of their intelligence but also because of other qualities they may possess.
- A wealthy, beautiful, emphatic, and intelligent woman might, for example, be a "goal" for the narcissist since the narcissist is always about what they want: a successful and intelligent woman might look like an extra source of income to the narcissist.
- The more successful an intelligent person is, the more they would look like objects to be captured by a narcissist, and it is natural for the narcissist to seek control of successful people so that they can have what they have.
- Past trauma conditions intelligent people into associating love with abuse
- It is also true for smart people, and also it doesn't apply to most intelligent people, but in some cases, victims of childhood traumas can carry their wounds into adulthood.
- When the wounds of past hurts are not healed, the intelligent adult often tolerates abusive behavior and confuse it with love.
- Human vulnerabilities have nothing to do with the rational mind.
- Narcissists since the voids in other peoples' lives and will come into the life of intelligent people like they came to fill the void.
- They do this with love bombing and showering intelligent people with great attention. A vulnerable person will read no ulterior motive behind the attention they receive, particularly if the narcissist comes into their lives at the point where they are not feeling hopeful, maybe because of the loss of a dear one or some other kind of misfortune.
- The problem with vulnerabilities is that even intelligent people might feel manipulated, but these rational feelings are ignored because the narcissist is filling a particular need or longing.

- Through degrading cycles of abuse, intelligent people may not realize that they are being tricked because their vulnerabilities may outweigh their intelligence.
- Gaslighting narcissists have a lifetime's worth of training.

Indeed, even the most intelligent people can fall victim when they meet a narcissist. In general, narcissists are enchanting individuals who can trick even judges, law enforcement authorities, and specialists.

Narcissists have always been the manipulators they are since childhood. Over time, they might refine their manipulative tactics, so they find it easy to capture them when they encounter intelligent people.

It is crucial to note that nobody is genuinely, ever invulnerable to being an abusive object for a narcissist. The narcissist will get their way with intelligent people with:

Twisted Truths

It is one of the most common ways that narcissists manipulate smart people. They either gloss over the truth, or they blatantly deny the truth. To get their needs met, it is shocking that they will go to any extent.

A narcissist will make a statement or a promise and deny it even in the same breath. They can pretend that the truth isn't what it is and conveniently put it on the smart people that it was an overreaction on their part, or a bad memory, or a need for unnecessary drama.

Guilt-Tripping

Another thing narcissist love to do when they are gaslighting and manipulating intelligent people is to lay guilt. Guilt is a go-to tactic many narcissists use without anyone realizing it. Guilt is very subtle, and many times, even people outside the gaslighting situation won't see it.

The narcissist might perform a subtle action or say a phrase or hold their body in a certain way to keep the victim in check-in social situations. It keeps the victim in a constant state of anxiety and fear. The narcissist will deny if anything concerning the awkward behavior comes up in an upcoming conversation.

Narcissists are good at making their victims believe they didn't experience what they did, or they made up something in their heads.

Kill the Messenger

Here is another thing narcissist do to gaslight and manipulate intelligent people: they ask smart people to "kill the messenger."

What does the phrase mean? Narcissists, as controlling individuals, tend to use other people as messengers or the mediators for some of the aspects of the victim's life.

Without concern for anyone involved, these abusive sets of humans will use various people to send victims hurtful messages or blame victims for their issues.

People will often walk up to the victims and state that they are concerned about the victim's problems and express themselves, so everyone passing by will hear them. It leads to people coming around the victim and trying to offer support in genuine ways.

Unknown to the intelligent victim, these concerned individuals are just playing their parts in a narcissist script.

So, what the narcissist is doing most, is to employ "messenger" people who mean well and have no malicious intent for the victim and tell them a lie that the victim is having a big problem. Of course, they are doing such things to deflect responsibility and further isolate and control their victims.

Passive Aggressiveness

Narcissists are infamous for loving the passive-aggressive manipulation tactic. They have a knack for hitting victims where it hurts, and they will find and exploit the weak spots of intelligent people, so it's easier to make them feel guilty. Of course, the narcissistic injury part comes in: the narcissist will then pretend to be the victim.

At the point of playing the victim, intelligent people feel sorry for them, and even if they don't feel ashamed and go with the narcissist's charade, the narcissist will cry and whine and moan act pathetic to get what they want.

They will use all means to accuse intelligent people of being abusers, insensitive, mean, and hateful. They project themselves onto the victim. People are just extensions and objects to narcissists, even the people who are the closest to them. They do not care. They're users who don't mind using their friends and other family members to get what they want and to hurt others.

Fear and Intimidation

The other tactic narcissists use on intelligent people is fear and intimidation. They might resort to anger and threats in their words to manipulate and intimidate the victim. They are good at using anger and fear to coerce the people in their lives. They use threats and angry outbursts to make victims feel uncomfortable and upset

Head Stepping

Another behavior a narcissist will use to manipulate you is what is called head stepping. A narcissist is very likely to belittle victims to try to bring them down to their level.

They are insecure people who feel threatened by intelligence and will use head stepping to make their victims wrong in other people's eyes. The main goal of head stepping is to make the victim feel inferior and more comfortable to control. They criticize you and tear down victims to make them feel inferior because it makes them feel superior.

Chapter 18. What Are the Possible Cures for Narcissist?

The most prominent cure for Narcissistic Personality Disorder is psychotherapy. Or in a more specific sense, talk therapy, also known as Psychodynamic Therapy or Psychoanalytic Therapy. This procedure allows a client to relate better to other people and gain the ability to form intimate and long-lasting relationships. Through talk therapy, a client can foster healing and growth so that life can become more enjoyable and rewarding. Psychotherapy is also the process of understanding the sources of the client's emotions. It includes his hidden drives, motives, and other unconscious factors.

Through talk therapy, the mental health professional will help the client realize his real potential compared to the possibilities and capabilities he has created in his fictional world. This process also increases the client's ability to understand, be aware, and regulate his emotions to avoid impulsivity and aggression towards the self and other people. Another distinguishing factor of Narcissistic Personality Disorder is their inability to take criticisms constructively. Through talk therapy, the client develops a sense of tolerance to the negativities and issues that can impact his feelings or self-esteem. This form of treatment also helps the client to release unwanted emotions and thoughts of insecurity and isolation. It makes a person realize that he doesn't have to phish for approval and affection because the right people will give it to him wholeheartedly. Talk therapy is essential to help the clients reach their goals through acceptable means in society to avoid their drive to undermine, insult, and underestimate other people's capabilities so that they can feel superior.

There are different approaches to psychotherapy that can help people with Narcissistic Personality Disorder. Besides talk therapy, we also have Behavioral Therapy, Cognitive Therapy, Humanistic Therapy, and Person-Centered Therapy.

Behavioral Therapy

This method is defined as changing what a person does to the help of a therapist. Behavioral theorists have proposed aversion therapy in which a behavior is paired with some form of punishment. The everyday use of this therapy is to help people quit substance abuse disorders. However, this can be used to help people with Narcissistic Personality Disorder. A behavioral psychologist might associate with punishment every time that client has behaved poorly in other people's eyes, such as insulting, demeaning, overdramatizing, and other actions done by people with NPD.

Behavioral Therapists also use desensitization, also known as the process of a gradual introduction of the stressful stimulus. As for people with Narcissistic Personality Disorder, a distress-causing motivation for them is imperfection, loneliness, lack of attention, and criticisms. To slowly change the perception of people towards these aspects, a gradual introduction could be used.

Cognitive Therapy

This form of therapy has been developed to help clients to change their self-defeating thought patterns and behavior. For a long time, cognitive behavioral therapy has been pro to help people with various psychological disorders.

One technique used for cognitive therapy is known as Cognitive Restructuring Techniques. This method aims to help people identify their thinking patterns responsible for their negative moods and effective behaviors. When these have been determined, the therapist will help the client foster new perspectives towards these adverse cognitive functions.

It helps assign more positive regard to the negative thinking patterns that cause disparaging behavior.

Another technique for successful cognitive therapy is known as Graded Exposure Assignments. In this method, the therapist will allow the client to be systematic and approach their greatest fears. It will enable the patients to deal with their anxiety and control their emotions during a very threatening situation. Your system at the exposure, the client starts to master these feared situations one-by-one, until he finally can control his feelings and thoughts as the event arises.

Activity scheduling is also a common way to help people increase the onset of behaviors that they should be doing more. In several cases of people with Narcissistic Personality Disorder, they should be interacting with people more. They should start to learn to work in a team so they can foster cooperativeness and responsibility. Through activities scheduling, and NPD client is taught to say sorry more and say thank you often. He or she needs to learn the etiquette on how to complement other people to avoid any narcissistic and selfish means of degrading people to feel better.

Another essential technique introduced by cognitive therapy is mindfulness. It is a technique they borrowed from Buddhism in which a person is taught to disengage from ruminating or obsessing about negative things. Mindfulness is also a way of how people can be aware of their reality. So, they can match their goals to their actual capabilities in place of success.

Humanistic Therapy

This form of therapy focuses on the person's nature rather than comparing his behavior experiences to others' similar problems. Humanistic therapy perceives the person as a whole, and it structures its foundation from the client's perspective himself, who is an active observant of his actions. Humanistic therapy is commonly used to treat people with personality disorders, depression, anxiety, addiction, and schizophrenia. Through this process, a person can reach his full potential by acknowledging his strengths rather than his weakness, searching for his purpose, and setting motivational goals.

Person-Centered Therapy

This form of therapy uses a non-authoritative approach that allows patients to have a more significant role during treatment. This approach aims to let the client create a solution on his or her own with just the psychotherapist's guidance. The therapist only acts as a compassionate facilitator who only listens to what the client has to say without any judgment. During the process, the therapist's objective is to encourage and support the client without interrupting or interfering with the client's self-discovery process. Through this method, the client game can acquire a stronger sense of identity, gain more self-confidence, and build healthy and worthwhile interpersonal relationships.

How to Handle NPD in Therapy

There are instances when clients are referred to a psychologist without their consent or their idea. Knowing that people with Narcissistic Personality Disorder see themselves as perfect, they will believe they do not need any psychological intervention. Heck, they do not acknowledge that they are mentally sick. During these cases, we need to learn how to handle patients like this to help us grow and heal from their abnormality. But how do we do it to patients with Narcissistic Personality Disorder during treatment?

According to some experts, to successfully handle a narcissist person before treatment, kiss up to that person and gain trust. Do this in the form of praise, affirmation, and approval. Compliments sound useful to them, especially when they observe that they have your full attention. As a psychologist, use this to your advantage. Keep on leaning towards them without saying anything about the purpose as to why they are brought to therapy. Narcissists love to talk about themselves. So, lure them into opening up about their childhood experiences or their difficulties as a child. Sooner, you will probably hit something sensitive, and they start to overdramatize. Then, employ the element of comfort. Tell them about the importance of their healing to get over these negative thoughts and experiences. Make them understand the importance of doing therapy for their good. You can tell them that undergoing treatment will allow them to achieve their dreams to make them feel better. Narcissists love to hear when they feel like they are taking advantage of the efforts of other people. But as you move on to the process of therapy, they will soon have values realizations about themselves and their reality. They might not show this at first because they have pride, but you will observe a gradual improvement of their attitude towards your approach in therapy. If the practitioner can advise, use the "What would people think?" approach. We all know that narcissists are preoccupied with the way people judge them. Ask them what people would think when they found out that the client has this kind of weakness. Please encourage them to receive help from you. But first, make them believe that you are not the kind of person who would use their information to ruin them. Narcissistic people can be very paranoid, so gain their trust. Approach them in a way that they would perceive you to be non-threatening to their ego. Pretend that you worship them, and you love what they do if you have to. But it should only be in the hopes of getting them to open up their inner thoughts to you. Show them a non-disclosure contract if need be and explain your duties and ethical code of conduct as a practitioner. Moving forward to the "What would people think" bait makes them believe that these weaknesses and insecurities may be used against them by other people. It is why they need to be fixed as soon as possible. It is where you start to introduce therapeutic methods to change their lifestyle and their cognitive processes. Soon enough, they will begin to show changes in behavior and personality.

Another cunning way to deal with the narcissistic person is through role-playing. Make them believe that a model is rewarded by doing something useful, like giving to other people and cooperating during teamwork. Make them realize that there are positive things that can happen when you do good deeds. In contrast, when a person keeps on demeaning and insulting people for their benefit, they can get punished. If possible, the model should be just like the client to identify with it. It could be an effective startup to ready the client for a change.

Whatever you do in dealing with your clients, always be patient and determined.

Keep an open mind and realize that all of that need help. You might be the only key for them to survive in this cruel world. It stresses you out when dealing with cases like these, especially Narcissistic Personality Disorder, which is considered as cancer in society. They can cause a terrible headache as they don't know how to acknowledge their disease. But remember that they are victims too. If the rules were reversed, wouldn't you want to be helped by other people when you have a severe medical condition? It is our job as a practitioner to provide competent service to different people. And to do this, we should commit to our societal obligations and do whatever we can to develop a service that our clients need.

However, there are times when a practitioner needs to terminate the client-therapy relationship. It would help if you endorsed the patient to another practitioner when your methods and treatments are not working anymore. To help the patients fulfill their highest potential, they need a practitioner who can provide what is best for them. If you know it within yourself that you cannot help the person in need, do not deny them the service. Instead, explain to them that they need to see another professional experience a more active recovery from the psychological illness. The downside is, this could be very difficult to take on the part of your client. It would be best if you gave the closure they need to start over with a new therapist.

Chapter 19. The Narcissist's Target

The victims of narcissistic abuse frequently share similar traits that mark them as easy to manipulate. While this may be unconscious on the narcissist part, they are attracted to a handful of features that are the most conducive to getting what he wants. When you understand what the narcissist values most in a target, you learn how to guard yourself and not fall victim due to your personality.

Codependent

Codependency is a sign of a dysfunctional relationship. It refers to people around a drug addict that enables continued addiction; it is also relevant about the narcissist. The codependent does not acknowledge that there are any problems in her relationship. She decides to disregard or ignore her own emotions and needs because focusing on herself has never been conducive to her relationship or having a good time. She has learned that walking on eggshells, catering to every whim of the other person, keeps the other person happy, which means she is safe. She lives in denial to survive and frequently completely detaches herself from situations around her to stay. She goes through the motions without really feeling. She walks through life and her relationship as a husk of a person, pouring every bit of herself into bettering the other person.

The narcissist loves the codependent because the codependent will put time into pleasing the narcissist. Her feeling of self-worth is entirely related to caring for others, to a fault. There is a small difference between compassionate and codependent. The codependent has taken her kindness to the extreme of martyring herself out for the narcissist's benefit. Her intentions are kind, but the mark is missed. The narcissist is enabled in his behaviors, believing that they are justified. It creates a destructive environment for the codependent that the narcissist thrives within.

Ultimately, the narcissist feels that the codependent is the ultimate target. The codependent already has low self-esteem, attempts to do things with good intentions, and has the intense desire to help those around her. The narcissist does not hesitate to take advantage of this person, knowing that he will more easily get what he craves, and the codependent never leaves because she sees no reason to.

Caregiver Personality

Similar to the codependent, but less extreme, the caregiver personality type is quite attractive to the narcissist. While this person may not necessarily have low self-esteem, he does have good intentions and the desire to care for another individual. The caregiver naturally wants to help other people. He sees everyone as deserving of love and help and would give the shirt off his back to someone to better the other person's experience. The caregiver is selfless and dedicated to improving the lives of those around him. He is patient and willing to put up with far more abuse or mistreatment than the average person because he believes that the other person deserves to be cared for. The compassionate, patient nature of the caregiver is precisely what the narcissist needs. She will think that this person will be willing to put in the effort to ensure that the narcissist is cared for. With some manipulation and action on the narcissist's part, she has the potential to be browbeaten into codependency. The narcissist craves someone dedicated to caring for her, and the caregiver is quite likely to do so.

Empathetic

Suitable targets for the narcissist are empathetic. Like the caregiver and codependent, those who are quite empathetic typically enjoy taking care of other people to ease their pain. The empath can feel the pain of other people so intimately it is as if she is the one being exposed to the cause of the problem herself, and she seeks to alleviate that pain in others. She does not want those around her to suffer in any way and will do whatever she can to help.

The narcissist knows this and knows that empaths are particularly in tune with their feelings. The narcissist can weaponize her empathy and use it against her, playing on guilt to keep her in line. He knows that the empath will be easy to manipulate because she is so susceptible to guilt trips. Empathy, being one of her best traits as an individual, becomes her weakness, and the narcissist takes advantage of it to better himself.

Has What the Narcissist Wants

It is not only times the narcissist will pick out a target that is not easily manipulated or controlled. She may see someone else with what she wants and choose to befriend them to learn their secrets or have some of their powerful benefits. She will likely mirror this person quite closely, mimicking their actions to learn from them. If she can get close to the person who has what she wants, she may get some by default. For example, imagine a narcissist who has befriended the mayor of a town. Any time she goes out with the mayor, she gets treated with similar prestige simply because she is in the mayor's company, and over time, her knowing the mayor may even raise her reputation in town. If people know she is close to the mayor, they may treat her better in hopes of her excellent word getting back to him, and she preys on this. She can use this to her advantage, and over time, she is eventually recognized in her small community as well, and she has done nothing but draw the mayor into believing they are friends.

Dysfunctional or Abusive Upbringing

Those who have grown up in dysfunctional or abusive environments often never learned what healthy or normal indeed looks like regarding relationships. They never learned how to identify when something is dangerous, abnormal, or worth avoiding. All of the abuse and dysfunction became the individual's normal, which means his or her tolerance for putting up with a narcissist's abusive, manipulative antics may be far beyond what it should be. The narcissist knows this and seeks to use it to his advantage. He knows that the one who grew up abused is not likely to understand what healthy relationships look like, and therefore, she will never understand what she is missing. She will assume whatever was modeled for her during childhood is normal and expected, thinking that there is nothing better beyond that.

For example, imagine you grew up with parents who hated each other's guts but could not afford to divorce while still sustaining the children. You grew up watching your parents argue and hate each other, disrespecting each other at every opportunity, and calling each other names regularly. Though you may know that your parents' relationship was not happy, you may struggle to dissociate that association with healthy relationships. You understand that they were not pleased, but you are almost destined to repeat those mistakes in your relationships, and would not think twice about a partner that may behave similarly. To you, they are not as alarming and foreign as they would be to someone who grew up with parents who doted on each other. The narcissist will take that tolerance and push it to the extreme, knowing it can only benefit him and his desires.

Nonconfrontational

Those who fear or avoid confrontation want to live a life free of conflict. They are typically quite easygoing, and the narcissist sees this relaxed nature and desire to live without fighting and decides to take advantage of it. The narcissist's manipulation tactics require her not to be called out when she attempts to control a situation. Those who hate conflict or confrontation are the most likely to avoid calling out the narcissist's antics. The nonconfrontational are far more likely to decide to give in to the narcissist's demands and suffer in silence than cause an issue, knowing that calling out the behaviors would result in exactly what the narcissist wants to avoid. It becomes a situation in which the nonconfrontational person has to decide between being miserable and not calling out the abuse or being miserable after calling out the abuse and inviting more of it.

The narcissist understands this tendency to avoid conflict and seeks out people who will not fight back. He takes advantage of the person who avoids confrontation only because it betters his situation.

Low Self-Esteem and Lack of Confidence

Both low self-esteem and low confidence lead to easily manipulated people, as both people crave love, but feel as though they are unworthy or undeserving of it. They feel as though they are impossible to love, seeing their flaws as their entire identity instead of just a small part of who they are. The narcissist knows this; the narcissist often seeks to break down other people's self-esteem solely because those with lower self-esteem are easier to manipulate. If possible, the narcissist will strictly go for someone with low self-esteem because she wants to get what she wants with the little effort. If the narcissist has targeted already feels terrible about himself, he will be easier to manipulate. The work is already half-finished, and all the narcissists will have to do is add the finishing touches to groom the individual into whatever she wants.

Chapter 20. Narcissists and Sex

When a narcissist is seeking sexual pleasure, they put on a typical act of charisma to win you over. They can be compared to salespeople in this respect because they make you trust them on a level where you will be eating out of their hands. They are such masters at this art by using heavy flirting, downright over the top flattery, and subtle persuasion to get what they want in the end.

They continue the manipulations by luring you to the bedroom shortly after your first date to impress you and then entrap you in their web. There are people out there who are naturally charming and excellent lovers. The difference with the narcissist is that they are not interested in creating a lasting bond with you in a meaningful way. You are merely there as an object to be used because you have something to offer that the narcissist craves.

It is part of the withholding manipulation that is a test to let the narcissist know where your boundaries stand. They can gauge how much under their thumb you are. They will then continue to dish out more manipulation tactics to garner even more control over you. You would be amazed at how much potential a person can have over someone in the bedroom and life in general.

Narcissists are always fishing for compliments to boost their egos, so they may ask you direct questions that would make you feel uncomfortable answering every time you have sex. They would be directly asking you if it was the best you ever had or how many orgasms you had. They may also ask you to go into explicit detail about every moment of the encounter. It may seem very strange as they were also there, but you must remember, they are not concerned about your experience. They are only looking for the praise and that they have gotten what they wanted from you.

Suppose you happen to say anything that they do not want to hear, such as perhaps you have had better or you start criticizing the experience negatively. In that case, there is undoubtedly going to be a backlash from the narcissist. It may happen in the way of a blown-up argument to scare you into never wanting to critique them negatively again. They can also use it as an attack on you personally, so they feel like they are still the dominant person in the situation.

Sex with a narcissist can also be very robotic, especially once the honeymoon period is over. Since the narcissists see themselves as a sort of ringmaster, they expect the show to go as planned in their heads. It means that they know exactly what positions or even specific phrases they want to hear from their partner during sex.

Because they control every aspect of the show, they have selected you specifically for the part, be it for your prestige, attitude, physical aspects, or a combination of all three. They care nothing about the deep connection and see you as objects they can manipulate to create the perfect experience in their eyes and for their pleasure.

They love to dominate the situation and even seek out submissive types to make it easier for them to have total control in the bedroom. It also bleeds into other areas of their partner's life as they can continue to manipulate every day to please them.

You may even have a narcissist that boasts about being game for anything, but these are likely just words. Narcissists are very self-conscious, and as a result, they want to look the best they can in bed. They may refrain from certain positions, so they do not look bad in any way. It leads to boredom in the bedroom as the narcissist will likely play out the same scenarios day after day because they enjoy that particular play of events.

They can also be particular when it comes to oral sex. It may demand that you perform oral sex for them regularly, but they will refrain from doing the same for you. When you have the same requests, they will most likely turn it around to perform what sexual acts they want at the time. If you start to refuse the sexual acts they want to perform because it is not something you enjoy, they will gaslight you into thinking that your wants and desires are wrong, even degrading you. It may also be when the narcissist asks for a particular dirty sexual act that you do not feel comfortable doing. To appease them, you follow through with their request, and then the narcissist may condemn you for performing the degrading acts, saying that it was your idea all along.

Sometimes it does work out that you have the same likes in and outside of the bedroom. Some people like the exhibitionist side of the narcissist who always has risky encounters, even breaking the law at specific points. When it comes to sex, it is all about the narcissist. The truth is you are there to satisfy their needs. They do not mind if you are enjoying yourself as long as they get theirs. This realization will start to come to you after the honeymoon period is over, and the true narcissist starts to make themselves known. You will then begin to feel the disconnection from the absence of real connection because of the narcissist's inability to display love as we have defined in society.

Self-absorbed narcissists may have several mirrors in the bedroom to watch themselves while performing sex, and they may enjoy taking videos or pictures of themselves to watch after. Many times, they will take these pictures without your consent. It also adds to the bedroom's disconnect as they will be paying attention to themselves more than you. It is also common for the narcissists to make comments on their breasts or penis' size and how wonderful they are. They will even ask you to compare them to your past lovers' breasts or penis so that they can compare and continue to inflate their sense of self.

Other than the emotional factor being non-existent in the sexual relationship with a narcissist, they devalue your individuality by dismissing your priorities, feelings, and thoughts. Sometimes they will ignore you or pretend to be listening when their mind is elsewhere.

It is common to get the cold shoulder emotionally or physically as soon as the sexual act has been completed. It can be in the way of falling asleep after hearing the praises of their stellar performance, physically leaving, or being devoid of emotional connection during the refractory period. It is also a tactic used to starve you of something that you crave if this was not done during the honeymoon period. They may go back and forth with this manipulation of supply and distance to make you need them more.

Because of the shallowness of the sexual acts, they do not make sense of commitment to any partner and are commonly found to cheat. If they don't take what they want from you, they will likely seek it from someone else who would be willing to give them what they want. It is incredibly easy for the narcissist because they have the skills to sweep certain types of people off their feet quickly, and they have no moral qualms about infidelity.

Sex sells in our society, and narcissists use this tool to their advantage. It has been said from narcissistic abuse victims that they did not want to leave violent situations because the sex was that good. It would also be coupled with the other manipulation and brainwashing techniques that would have the victim forget about the narcissist's negative instances. In turn, they would solely remember the ecstatic ways they made them feel during the good times, especially during sex.

The extensive you get into a relationship with a narcissist, the sex would end up being a form of addiction for the victim. It is a way of temporarily escaping the torment and pain that has become their life. Adversely, it can also be the cause of the problem. The dichotomy makes the relationship difficult to break because they are pacifiers, and the oppressor depends on each moment. Sometimes, these are felt simultaneously.

Certain neurochemicals are released in your body during sex, making one more vulnerable to the addiction of being with the narcissist. These include cortisol, dopamine, noradrenaline, and oxytocin. It is said that, as the narcissistic relationship, it can take from 18 to 22 months for your brain's chemical levels to return to normal.

Once they get you to the point where you cannot live without them, they will start to pull away. To make them come back to you, you begin to agree to their requests, no matter how wrong it is in your mind's eye. It will work for them to come back, but you will notice that they very rarely follow through with what they promised you. It is a lose-lose situation for the victim and narcissist as this is a cycle that is extremely hard to break once it gets to the point where the victim is chasing the narcissist. It has also been found that with a lack of sexual morality, narcissists will commit incest by sexually assaulting family members, including underage children. In the narcissist's eyes, they are doing nothing wrong, and some enjoy breaking the law. It soothes the adrenaline rush they crave so much. They also feel that children and family members can be more vulnerable, making them a perfect target for control and manipulation. The sexual deviancy and abuse are another power mechanism used by narcissists to control the situation. They can exercise this power over their partners by having them go into explicit detail about their past lovers, usually saying that it is a turn-on for them or any other explanation for you to feel comfortable talking about these instances. They will then use these past experiences you have had to degrade and belittle you throughout the relationship. They can also be used afterward as a blackmailing tool to get you to come back or to engage in vengeful, hurtful acts.

On the reverse side of things, when the relationship gets to the vengeful side, the narcissist will start putting their lover down by saying they will never be better than the other lovers they have had in the past. When it gets to this point, some narcissists enjoy hurting their partners emotionally, making them feel superior.

Chapter 21. Three Types of Empathy

Empathy is thus rather beneficial. However, in cases where an empath cannot cope with all the feelings and emotions received and precepted from others, empathy may feel like a burden too heavy to withstand alone.

Take a look at the types of empathy and try to find yourself in description and definition:

Cognitive Empathy

Cognitive empathy is strictly related to the theory of mind, as referred to by psychologists and behavioralists. Cognitive empathy carries the ability to understand others by understanding their mental state and their mindset. Empaths with increased cognitive empathy can somewhat predict what the other person would say based on an understanding of their mind and character. Cognitive empathy draws roots from the ability to deduct what the other person might say or think based on their last "performance" as perceived by a cognitive empath. Psychologists refer to this social ability as to "thinking about thinking," where the empath with this ability concludes what the other person is thinking or is capable of, based on determining their mindset, mental state, knowledge, emotions, desires, and even beliefs. It is not only that cognitive empathy allows you to guess what others might think, but it also enables you to understand why is that so – why is someone doing what they are doing based on all factors that you can perceive. Cognitive empathy represents a rather valuable social skill.

It is referred to as "the theory of mind" because as a person with strong cognitive empathy. You may only presume or predict what the other person would say or what the other person thinks or can do based on what you know about them and their personality, making it a theory more than a fact. Cognitive empathy is otherwise rather useful as a social skill as it may help you generate an appropriate social response based on what you perceive within your mind theory. Cognitive empathy is a rather crucial aspect of our social interaction. As we mature, we can nurture and improved at an early age when your mind and emotions are yet to be defined and developed alongside your character and personality. As we grow up and maturing, understanding other people's mental state becomes very important about responding to other people's actions and reactions. Cognitive empathy helps us understand how someone's mental state may influence their actions. Resolving conflicts with other people also requires understanding how others might feel and how others may act based on their personality and various factors related to their mind and emotions.

Affective Empathy

Affective empathy is perhaps a type of empathy that may take the best out of an empath if you are not sure how to respond to the way you feel about other people's emotions. The definition of affective empathy states that this type of empathy represents the ability to understand how others think so that you can act by their feelings. This sensitivity can also backfire as an empath who has increased affective empathy might be physically affected by what others feel. While sympathy and compassion allow us to associate with other people and express our understanding of other people's emotions. By being there for them and providing emotional and mental support, affective empathy affects empaths to feel the same way others do once they get emotionally involved. This state relates to the case as a product of emotional experiences that don't belong to us but can be mirrored by our brain receptors, where the brain creates a personal response to other people's distress. The way it would generate an emotional reaction in case you would be the one going through that same situation someone else is going through. That is how effective empathy makes an empath feel the same way the other person does while also carrying the ability to handle others' emotions as their emotional distress. Still, affective empathy is yet another type of empathy that represents a social skill, as it allows us to feel concerned for other people based on the emotions we perceive.

Somatic Empathy

Somatic empathy relates to feeling physical effects triggered by how you perceive that other people think. With somatic empathy, an empathic body may have a physical reaction to an emotion that other people are experiencing. For instance, as an empath who has increased somatic empathy, you may feel nervous when you notice that someone else feels the same way, or even when you know that the person you are connecting with is anxious about something. The same goes for any feeling; somatic empathy represents the ability to physically experience other people's emotions, which can also be somewhat overwhelming for empaths who cannot control how they experience other people's feelings. The somatic nervous system would make the same response to other people's experiences, just as it would be the case if you were the one going through that specific case, which is how somatic empathy is defined. Regardless of which type of empathy is more vital, experiencing other people's emotions physically and emotionally may be exhausting for empaths who give in, or better said, "feel in," which is the exact definition of the word "empathy" derived from the German word Einfühlung. Empathy is a term that has been studied for around a century by far; however, the word empathy can also find its origins in the Greek word empatheia, roughly translated to "in feeling."

How Can We Benefit from Empathy and Why Is It Important?

What needs to be understood is that empathy is indeed a crucial social skill and should be present in every human being. They don't care how others feel, leading to isolation and psychosocial deviations. After all, we are social beings, which means that we rely on others' company just as much we would be unable to survive without being connected to at least one person. Since early ages, when we are still growing up and learning, we also learn how to behave around other people and how to be able to generate an adequate social or emotional response when it is noted that there is a lack of appropriate reactions. For example, two children are playing, and they are not getting along well because they both like the same toy at the same time. As they are yet growing up, they don't understand the concept of making compromises and may even have problems with sharing as little children are often acting selfishly. Both children are crying, but neither of them can understand how the other well as their empathy is yet to be developed. It is where an adult has to balance everything and explain how the two children should act appropriately. There is an exclusion to every rule, so there are children whose character will allow them to empathize already at an early age even though social skills might not be entirely developed at that point. This child usually grows up to be highly sensitive to other people's emotions, which can sometimes be harmful to their good.

Talking about the importance of empathy, you also need to note that some people may use their empathy as understanding how other people feel to manipulate those people. Empathy is thus a crucial part of the way we connect with others and the way we connect.

The way we connect through empathy is a benefit that comes hand in hand with this social skill. People can empathize with others, but we can even experience emotions of fictional characters we see in movies and books, which allows us to experience emotions that we otherwise wouldn't be able to, making empathy an essential part of emotional intelligence.

What is important to you to know as a highly sensitive being that has an increased capacity of feeling what other people think, is that despite occasional hardships that may arrive with overreacting to what others are feeling, empathy is truly a gift. That gift allows us to be what we are born to be – human beings that can connect and coexist most poetically – by feeling other people's emotions, which altogether describes the role and importance of empathy.

Precisely thanks to empathy, you can create bonds and healthy relationships with others, can connect on an emotional level, understand others, and understand your own emotions and how these emotions affect your actions.

How Empathy May Affect Empath's Everyday Life?

As we emphasized more than once, empathy is a crucial social skill that helps us establish relationships with other people and connect by understanding our own emotions and other people's emotions. Being an empath is healthy and even necessary based on that definition. But, what about the case of overactive empathy?

How to tell if you are being overactive in empathizing to the extent where your empathy is negatively affecting your everyday life?

There are signs that you may pick up in your reactions to other people's emotions by that may indicate that you might be an overactive empath, which may harm you mentally, spiritually, and psychologically.

Some people are sensitive to how others feel, which can sometimes go beyond their control, which is why protecting themselves from the negative influence of other people's emotions comes in as a crucial point of survival. Since you have come this far with the book, you are probably having a hard time balancing the effects that different people leave on you with their own emotional experiences that are quickly soaked in by your sensitive nature. That is how empathy may affect your everyday life, leaving you stranded on protecting yourself from harmful effects that different emotional experiences may imprint on your emotions map. Starting from feeling overwhelmed to feeling physically exhausted, the inability to control the effects that empathy may be leaving on, you may make your life far more difficult.

To the point where overactive empathy feels like a curse, which is less likely the case with people who can balance the way they are receiving and perceiving different emotional experiences that don't originally belong to them.

Chapter 22. Codependency and Narcissists

Codependency and narcissism are two sides to the same coin. They both lack a healthy sense of self, and they both struggle with defining who they are, bringing a whole barrage of issues to the table. Ultimately, codependency and narcissism are two different reactions to similar situations. Whereas the narcissist learns to be overtly selfish, the codependent learns to be overtly selfless. However, they are not always strictly opposites.

In some cases, the two can overlap to some degree. Someone can exhibit codependent behaviors in certain situations while behaving narcissistically in other contexts. For example, someone could be very codependent in a marriage or relationship, seeking to cater to their spouse's every whim, but be quite narcissistic with other people, such as friends or strangers. Though narcissism and codependence are both quite different, their root cause is the same.

What is Codependency?

In many normal relationships, we develop dependent relationships. It means that we prioritize our partners and rely on each other for love, and in times we need support. The connection is mutually beneficial, and neither person worries about expressing their real emotions. In a dependent relationship, both people can enjoy time spent away from the relationship while still meeting each other's needs.

However, in a codependent relationship, he feels that his only worth comes from being needed. He will make huge sacrifices, martyring himself out to ensure that the other person's needs are met. He only feels worthy if he can be needed. He exists solely for the relationship and feels as though he is worthless outside of that relationship. The relationship is his only identity, and he will cling to it at all costs, and within that relationship, he will ignore his own needs and wants, feeling as though they are unimportant.

Someone with codependent tendencies will struggle to detach from his partner because his entire sense of self is wrapped up in aiding that other person. It may get so bad that it begins to impact the codependent's life negatively. The codependent relationship can become all-consuming, taking over the person's life in all areas. Other relationships can weaken and fail as the codependent focuses solely on the person with which the relationship is held. Career potential may be lost, or the codependent may be fired when the relationship interferes with the work quality. Everyday responsibilities may be neglected in favor of catering to the enabler, the person with whom the codependent is in a relationship. Overall, the entire relationship is built on the faulty ground and is dysfunctional.

Causes of Codependency

Like NPD, many external factors are believed to cause a codependent personality to develop. Both codependency and narcissism are similar personality flaws, stemming from the same root cause of damaged self-esteem.

Poor Parental Relationships

Often, people who have developed a codependent personality have grown up repeatedly having conflicts with their parents throughout childhood. Their parents may have prioritized themselves, or somehow otherwise denied that the child's needs were essential. By downplaying the child's needs, the child internalizes that those needs are not important enough to meet. Due to all the time spent focusing on the parent's needs, the child never develops the independence and identity necessary to succeed in life. Feeling incomplete when not needed, these people frequently seek out other enablers that will allow them to continue living in this fashion.

Living with Someone Dependent on Care

When a child grows up around someone else who requires regular or around-the-clock care beyond the realm of normal, whether due to severe illness, injury, or some mental illness, the child's needs may go unmet in favor of meeting more pressing ones. As the child is pushed aside in favor of the person who needs the care, the idea of the child's needs become less-essential to become internalized. The child may engage in some care for the dependent person, causing his needs to be put on the back burner as he takes care of the person who literally cannot care for herself. While living with a family member who requires extra care does not necessarily cause codependency to develop independently.

Key Features of Codependency
Often, codependency manifests in incredibly recognizable ways. Though every person is different, and the behaviors will change depending on the relationship, there are several behavioral patterns associated with codependency. Knowing how to identify these will enable you to recognize when you or someone you know is exhibiting codependent tendencies. If you feel that you may be codependent, seeking a trained psychologist's professional opinion would be a great place to start on your journey toward understanding yourself.

Exaggerated Sense of Responsibility: Codependents frequently feel as though the weight of their loved one's actions is on their shoulders. They think they are directly in charge of the actions of their partners, children, or anyone else with which they are codependent.

Confuse Love and Pity: Codependents think that pitying and desiring to help someone is the same as love. They believe that they are doing it out of love every time they feel compelled to rescue someone instead of compassion for another human being.

Doing More Than Their Fair Share: Codependents tend to bear the burden of work, even when the share is more than unfair. They feel as though they have to take responsibility to support their enabler, even when it may be harmful to the codependent to take that added burden.

Sensitive When Good Deeds are Unrecognized: When a codependent feels as though her efforts have gone ignored, she is likely to feel hurt or as though she was not good enough. She will try to martyr herself further to get the recognition she craves to soothe her low self-esteem and prove that she matters.

Feeling Guilty When Caring for Self: Any time the codependent engages in acts she may see as selfish or unnecessary in the grand scheme of things, she will feel guilty. Her needs should be met last, and if not, she is behaving selfishly, which is unacceptable to her.

Rigid: Codependents do not tolerate change. They often seek out familiar things for this reason, which leads them to continually seek out other enablers in relationships, even if those enablers prove to be abusive.

Cannot Set Healthy Boundaries: Codependents see no boundaries between themselves and their enablers. They have no sense of self that is outside of the relationship or apart from the enabler. Because they fail to set boundaries, the relationship eventually consumes their lives and leaves little room for anything else. This lack of limits also leads to needs going unmet.

Needs Recognition to Feel Whole: Without recognition for good deeds and caring for others, codependents feel unwanted and unimportant. They require people to recognize their actions to help bolster their fragile self-esteem.

Need to Control Others: Codependents, feeling utterly responsible for the actions of their enablers, also seek some level of control over the relationships. Because the codependents always do everything possible for the enablers, they develop that control they desire, and the enabler allows them to have it. Without power, the codependents feel unable to help.

Fear of Abandonment: With their sub-par self-esteem and feeling as though they have no sense of identity beyond their relationship, codependents are terrified of being abandoned. They will do anything to keep the relationship going.

Poor Decision-making Skills: Frequently, their dysfunctional opinions and views of their relationships make the codependents make bad decisions. These could range from refusing to leave a dangerous situation because they want to stay with their partner or refuse to meet their needs, even if it makes them sick or hurt.

Difficulty Communicating: Codependents struggle to communicate their own needs and wants because they are so caught up in the idea that they do not matter. Even if they hate something, they will refuse to say it if they think it would be detrimental, even slightly, to the other person.
Unhealthy Dependence on Relationship: Codependents exist solely for their relationships and enablers, and that dependence on their enablers crosses the line into the territory of dysfunction.
Untrusting: Often, due to so much dysfunction in childhood, codependents tend to distrust those around them, especially those who insist that their needs should be met or that try to point out that their relationship is unhealthy.
Confrontation-Avoidant: Codependents avoid confrontation at all costs. They have developed their tendency to avoid their own needs due to avoiding confrontation, and that tendency to avoid confrontation has extended well into adulthood. The codependent will do anything to avoid a conflict, especially with the enabler.

Codependents and Narcissists

They meet every line on the narcissist's guide to choosing a target, and they are the ultimate victim for the narcissist. In their partnership, the codependent gives endlessly to the narcissist, who needs the attention to feel loved. The narcissist gets to provide the codependent with the gift of being needed. Both the narcissist and the codependent get their dysfunctional needs met. While this may seem like the perfect arrangement, it still encourages two people to live incredibly unhealthy lives. The codependent never has basic needs met and even has broken self-esteem and lacks an identity. The narcissist never gives back in the relationship and delves that the narcissist is the only one that matters. The narcissist's self-esteem and disordered thinking are not fixed through being catered to. It leads to an interesting relationship in which both the narcissist and the codependent enable each other.

Furthermore, this relationship leads to the codependent wanting to live through the narcissist. Over time, these patterns may lead to resentment, but the codependent will continue trekking through the relationship, martyring her to him because that is what she feels is the right thing to do. The narcissist typically will begin to exploit the codependent more and more over time, seeking out more narcissistic supply. The codependent eventually reaches a point of giving up, but despite this, neither partner is likely to leave. The narcissist loves the easy access to narcissistic supply and having someone willing to cater to his every whim. The codependent wants to feel needed, even though there is no appreciation reciprocated. Even if the relationship teeters toward abusive, the relationship becomes even more toxic and dysfunctional.

Chapter 23. The Narcissist and Psychological Games

Narcissists are very good at initiating dramatic psychological games, often at your expense. They can stir up conflict between you and other people, and once you are at each other's throats, they'll pretend they had absolutely nothing to do with the situation at hand. So, if you sense that a narcissist is playing some mind game intending to get you to react aggressively, you should take a step back.

Narcissists play games and start drama because they enjoy the chaos that ensues due to their machinations. When a narcissist starts a conflict between two people, he/she feels a sense of superiority over them — it feels like he/she is the puppet-master. You and others are tiny puppets ready to rip each other apart while he/she plays god over your lives. Before you fall into the trap that the narcissist sets for you, and find yourself tangled in a drama whose origin you can't even remember, let's look at some of the familiar games that a narcissist may try to get you involved in.

One typical game that narcissists play is the "emotional ping pong" game. It is where a person avoids taking responsibility for their actions by throwing that responsibility back to you. If the narcissist has done something reprehensible, instead of reflecting on their activities and admitting wrongdoing, they will throw the ball back at you somehow. They could try to blame you, shame you, project fault onto you, or even outright deny doing something wrong, making you seem crazy for even pointing it out. If you care about them, you might find yourself believe the lie and even making excuses on their behalf.

Narcissists always love to play different 'game' variations to make you seem crazy in front of other people. A narcissist could do something that indicates to you that they have malicious intent. Still, when you confront them, they can accuse you of having an overactive imagination, feigning innocence, or they can turn it around by accusing you of malice.

They could even get everyone around you to turn against you by making outrageous public accusations. Once you fall into that trap, you will start spinning out of control, trying to prove to others that you are right, but that will only serve to demonstrate the narcissist right. You have to learn to avoid reacting dramatically to a narcissist's actions, and you have to be able to tell when you are being set up.

The most infuriating game that narcissists play is "gaslighting." It is where the narcissist flatly denies remembering something that you know perfectly well that happened, and they insist that their memory is perfect and that you are the one who is mistaken. It is a dangerous game, and it is surprisingly common in abusive relationships. Suppose you stay for long with someone who "gaslights" you in the end. In that case, you will start doubting your perception of reality, and you will lose trust in your recollection of events, your reasoning, and intuition, and you will become a sitting duck for the abusive narcissist.

You have to remember to let the narcissist's games roll off your back because if you internalize everything that the narcissist tries to do to you, if you fall into every trap he sets for you, if you give in and react dramatically, in the end, you will lose.

If you play the narcissist's game for a long time, ultimately, you will suffer what pop-psychologists refer to as "death by a thousand cuts." It is where the narcissist will harm you in small ways over and over again until, in the end, they can wreck you. If you play the narcissist's games, he will destroy every part of you by disparaging your accomplishments, destroying your ego and your confidence, casting doubt on your values and your belief system, and dampening your soul. If you let a narcissist have their way, they will turn everything you are doing into a failure. If you are in a relationship, they will blame everything that goes wrong and takes credit for everything that goes right.

Don't engage in the narcissist's drama. Don't play games. As a decent person, you will be inhibited by your rationality and your sense of decency. The narcissist won't play by any rules, so you can be sure that you will lose. To win with a narcissist is to avoid playing their games altogether.

You don't need to justify yourself to the narcissist. When you interact with a narcissist, they will insist that you explain specific actions and choices that you have taken. You have to remember that your decisions are in your own best interests, and you don't owe the narcissist any explanation. Once you bother to explain yourself to the narcissist, it opens the door for them to then plant the seed of doubt on the decision that you have made to make you second guess yourself so that they can regain control over you. By all means, don't explain yourself. Let the narcissist know that you have already decided and not seek their input on the matter. It may seem not nice, but it's necessary.

You can be sure that the narcissists will keep pushing for you to explain things to them. The only way to win a narcissist's game is to avoid playing it altogether. Still, once you take the bait and explain an action you have taken or a decision you have made, the narcissist will come up with a hundred different questions and observations, all of which are tailor-made to diminish your conviction. They will tell you it's not in your best interest to do what you are doing, you are not smart enough or strong enough to do it, or you need their help to see your plan through. The narcissist knows that when you start doubting your perceptions and your convictions, you will have to rely on their guidance a lot more, giving them control over you. When you get to the point where you don't trust your judgment, you will accept the narcissist's ruling, and they will be able to tell you what to do and how to think and act at all times.

We will pinpoint some of the signs that can indicate to you that you are being gaslighted so that you are in a better position to stop doubting yourself and avoid further manipulation. First, the narcissist will start by telling a blatant lie. Since this is a person you have known for a while and you trust to some level, the lie will throw you off balance, and you will start doubting apparent things. The narcissist will then deny things that they said, even if you can prove that they did. The more vehement their denial, the more you question your reality!

The narcissist succeeds in gaslighting you because he wears you down over time. It's easy to think that you are too smart to get gaslighted, but the fact is that it doesn't happen instantaneously, it happens gradually, and one day you will wake up and find that you are so far gone. The way it works is that the narcissist will tell a small lie, stick with it and make you question your reality a little bit, but then you will decide that it's too tiny a lie to matter, so you will let it slide. The lies will then escalate both in magnitude and in frequency, and since you let the first one slide, you will have an easy time doing the same with the subsequent lies, until you get to the point where it's a norm. So, it would help if you didn't second guess yourself or let an obvious lie slide for even a second. Don't let the narcissist desensitize you to their lies.

Narcissists have perfected the art of turning things around to make it sound like you were the selfish one when it's clear that they are taking advantage of you. While you are still confused, trying to decipher what they are doing will make great strides towards altering your whole reality. They will also send confusing signals by occasionally acknowledging some of your claims so that you begin to think that perhaps you were mistaken about the rest of the claims. For example, if you accuse the narcissist of 3 different things, they could cap to one and then deny the other 2, and this makes you think that they might be credible to some extent.

While gaslighting and other forms of manipulation can be infuriating and confusing, they are surprisingly easy to fall for, so you have to be vigilant. Your best bet is to stick to your guns and hold on to your reality. Don't let anyone talk you out of decisions you have made, and by all means, don't ever substitute your perception for someone else's.

Chapter 24. Narcissism and Addiction

It's common for someone diagnosed with Narcissism Personality Disorder to have a co-occurring addiction to drugs or alcohol. The connection is likely due to the way the two coping mechanisms serve as ways to escape reality. Alcohol and drug use can allow a person to suppress or ignore negative and shameful feelings, just as a false persona can.

Narcissistic Personality Disorder can produce feelings of isolation because connecting with peers is extremely difficult. Addiction can have a similar effect. A person with NPD and an addiction might find that one disorder feeds the other. Narcissism and addiction, when co-occurring, must both be treated. The combination tends to make it extremely difficult for a patient to adhere to treatment. Drug and alcohol use can hamper any positive strides made in NPD treatment, delaying a patient's progress. Treatment for Narcissistic Personality Disorder is already a long, arduous process; substance abuse can substantially decrease its effectiveness. A comprehensive treatment plan is necessary to help a person discover underlying causes, build coping skills, and improve relationships.

Signs of Addiction

Sometimes, it can be challenging to know if you or a loved one has a substance abuse problem. Some typical symptoms are:

- Intense cravings to use a substance
- Interference with responsibility (work, school, home, etc.)
- Continued use despite negative consequences

- Developed tolerance to a substance
- Many unsuccessful attempts to discontinue use
- A substantial amount of time devoted to purchasing, using, and recuperating
- Use in dangerous situations.
- Awareness of but disregard to harmful effects
- Withdrawal symptoms upon stopping usage
- Using to avoid or abate withdrawal symptoms
- More significant quantities consumed than initially intended
- Higher frequency of usage than initially intended

Similarities

For someone in treatment for Narcissistic Personality Disorder, drug use or alcohol abuse can hinder the patient's ability to find success. Addiction and NPD are challenging to treat; when they are intertwined, treatment is typically more intensive.

The use of illegal substances can exacerbate symptoms of Narcissistic Personality Disorder. For example, feelings of irreproachability and superiority can become even more inflated, while levels of empathetic capabilities decrease even further.

A narcissist is consumed by how others view him or her. Optics are so essential that a narcissist might choose alcohol over other substances because it's more socially acceptable. Accessibility is seldom an issue, and a person with NPD can self-medicate with alcohol while being the friendly center of attention. Accordingly, a narcissist might choose to use marijuana for the same reasons.

Stimulants are also commonly used by people with NPD, possibly because the increased energy level can boost self-confidence. Stimulants (cocaine, Adderall, ecstasy, methamphetamine, Ritalin, etc.) allow a narcissist to increase productivity, which helps fulfill the need to uphold an appearance of success.

Substance abuse does not cause Narcissistic Personality Disorder. Many NPD tenets align with the criteria for a substance use disorder, and symptoms for each can mimic symptoms for the other. When addiction and Narcissistic Personality Disorder coincide, they can be challenging to differentiate.

The Cycle

The narcissistic abuse cycle can be integrated into the process of addiction. Once a narcissist feels threatened by criticism, they start to feel angry and then project that anger onto a victim. If the victim's response doesn't involve praise and validation, a narcissist might turn to his or her addiction. While the narcissist indulges in substance use, the victim will distance himself or herself. It confuses and insults the narcissist, so the cycle begins again.

Recovery

Before the recovery process, he or she must acknowledge the problem. This step is particularly challenging because someone with NPD sees himself or herself as above all others. Reluctance to admit the issue, combined with having someone "inferior" call attention to it, can lead to volatility. This first step can be complicated.

A true narcissist will want to undergo treatment at a superior facility where they will likely expect to be entitled to special treatment and impunity. Group therapy is designed to have people learn from one another, but a narcissist will be utterly disinterested in listening to others talk about themselves. Rehabilitation for substance abuse should be when a person devotes to the healing process. Still, a narcissist will most likely spend that time complaining, blaming others, and looking for an escape clause. Generally, the prognosis can be substandard if a narcissist allows illusions of grandeur to interfere with growth and learning during treatment.

The recovery process requires time, patience, and work. A narcissist is typically quite impatient, and recovery from addiction is not an overnight action. He or she will likely expect immediate, miraculous results; furthermore, the mentality is that his or her "elite" status will affect extraordinary change in a concise amount of time.

A narcissist is likely to want to eliminate addiction if he or she believes it is detrimental to the image they want to maintain. It's quite remarkable that a narcissist can sometimes abruptly discontinue substance use without being emotionally affected by busy it. Resuming the behavior in a while is usually a narcissist's way of proving that they are in control.

Dealing with a Narcissistic Addict

Substance use and addiction bring additional challenges to dealing with a narcissist. Both narcissistic and addictive behavior is inherently selfish, and entangling the two magnifies the destructive abuse that follows. A narcissist's arrogant mindset can create a dangerous situation. It is entirely impossible to convince someone that they have a problem with addiction if they refuse to acknowledge it. Living with a narcissistic addict can be overwhelmingly exhausting.

It's possible for friends and family to (sometimes unintentionally) enable narcissistic and addictive behaviors. A narcissist needs both to uphold his or her false self-image. Someone who fosters their narcissism will likely encourage the superiority complex while diminishing any substance use symptoms. A narcissist is very skilled at wearing masks; if a loved one doesn't see any visible signs of addiction, they can unknowingly support a habit, financially or otherwise. It is also easy for a narcissist's victim to fall into the role of an enabler. A narcissistic addict will tell a victim that he or she merely imagines substance abuse. Additionally, he or she might place blame for addiction on the victim. A narcissistic addict will manipulate a victim into thinking that their words and actions have caused, and continue to push, the abuser to self-medicate.

A large part of being supportive involves having reasonable expectations for a narcissistic addict throughout their recovery process. Clear and consistent boundaries are necessary for everyone involved.

Chapter 25. Narcissist Personalities

Narcissism comes in various forms. A narcissist can be a love partner, Father, mother, child, or another close person. In whichever way they come, narcissists can be bothersome and toxic. They create ugly experiences with the people around them. A child who experienced Narcissism from their parents at an early age tends to adapt and grow to become malignant narcissists. Also, they can fail to take and grow up as people with very low self-regard.

It is possible to experience Narcissism in more than one form, from more than one person. A person who grew up under the control of narcissistic parents can also find themselves under a narcissist partner's manipulations. Some of the people sometimes fall to the extreme and experience post-traumatic disorders or narcissism disorders.

Narcissistic Partner

When you meet a narcissist partner, you can easily find yourself into their love bomb due to their sweet words, the right approach, and even their helpful enticement tricks. This love bombing entails practicing overwhelmed signs of love. The kind of attraction you attract one another always reflects an excellent relationship. Note that, while the bomber was spending most of your time with this narcissistic partner, you seem not to identify the inner feelings.

Narcissistic partners always enjoy their relationships; you enjoy associating yourself with one another. The question remains, why do you feel like excluding yourself from such links? It is advantageous to the narcissists; they will use to take your weakness to strengthen your relationship with the abuser. Therefore, Love bombs are proofs to develop trust with your lover within a relationship. It could be compliments, romance, or even flattery, future premises, among others. Remember always to control yourself, or else the narcissist's abusers will manage all of your trust, honesty, and even love strength.

Moreover, these narcissists abusers can manipulate you and come up with exact things they intend to take from you. Furthermore, narcissists always plan to change out your outfit appearance in the relationship. You will now be forced to cope up with their way of doing things.

Remember that when you don't have 100% on your relationship partner, you highly make them very angry, they can even develop emotional feelings against you. They will not listen to your proposals, nor yet they won't create a good association with you. They will be just considering you as an ordinary person who does not add any positive value to their lives. Alternatively, love relationship always benefits them when they plan to remain intensely focus for a long time. Failing to meet this, you will be left hunting, failing to understand what you can do in those annoying situations.

Ways of differentiating real love expression using the exact actions in a relationship with your love partner

You will find it challenging to contrast a real from a fake one. Here is the main issue which will enable us to identify genuine love partners. You may find it very difficult to identify out when this was happening to you.

Narcissist Father

Narcissist's parent is the individual fathers who have influenced by Narcissistic Personality Disorder. They tend to stay too close to their children typically. These narcissists get shocked by how their children grow on their own. They always tend to be much busy with other unnecessary things. It gives it to them to worry about how other people think about their perspective.

This kind of Narcissistic parenthood mostly affects physical development; it affects their reasoning and emotional growth. They take much of their time to think about how their father has neglected their responsibilities, why their father has poor mental behavior on them.

Signs for a Narcissistic Father

You may have a different perspective in showing your father signs of Narcissism. Here are some of the characters which will lead you to know the real narcissistic father:

They Show Ignorance

A narcissist's father cannot stand criticism. He is against people who tried to point out his mistakes. Moreover, he cannot even listen to other people's ideas; they consider their final thoughts. They monopolize every conversation. What they say is essential; anything else said by another person does not matter to them. A narcissist father finds it difficult to identify with the needs of their children and incredibly emotional needs. They cannot share in the joy and sadness of their loved ones. They either show complete ignorance of others' requirements or take advantage of them to benefit themselves.

As talked about earlier, the narcissist tends to bring others down. They couldn't care less where it is due. There is fix darkness and confusion to a very shining star to remain on top and feel special. It makes them ignore and criticize their counterparts.

They Take Advantage of Others

This kind of Dad can use others to meet his needs. Having no empathy for others, they never care how their toxic behavior can affect other people. A narcissist father is capable of celebrating when their children has problematic issues. In this, they find a chance to take advantage of the problems, act heroic, and pretend they are helping and, in return, put their children under total manipulations.

He exploits the rights of other people to meet his needs. Always demanding and trying to manipulate. Expects favors that he doesn't deserve. The hard part about it is that their demands are unrealistic. They expect too much and give too little. Even the little they offer, to them that is a baited investment, they know that they will benefit and get back what they provide in the future.

Given a chance, narcissistic people can use other people like they have no value of themselves. They chew you up to the last bit of it; they destroy to conquer. When you fall for a narcissist, they steal your sense and make you believe that you are nothing without them. At this point, you keep on following them, and they mercilessly squeeze you until there is nothing left of you.

They Appear Scary

The different moods and feelings of this Dad always take many people to run away from them. The frightening rage cannot suit many of them. His anger can also make you run far away and never plan to meet him again. The narcissist father is easily provoked. One point, you are laughing with them, and then, they are on your neck. Criticism is one thing that makes them release their rage to the fullest. One has to walk on eggshells when dealing with such kind of a parent.

When they are angered, it means that something has injured their untouchable ego. Lowering their ego is something that this kind of person doesn't do. Hence, at the cage of their anger, they never think twice about doing anything to prove themselves. It can sometimes be dangerous to the victim. Cases are heard whereby a father hits badly or even kill his biological child because of a heated misunderstanding. It is always advisable to find the way out and away from the ranges of a narcissist.

They Seem to Be Perfect

A narcissist father is not all that bad. They have some advantages. In their battle to appear the ideal man, it is possible to benefit. You need to take the exact thing you are supposed to take from him. He is capable of providing you with the requirements. Narcissistic Father always gives excellent care to their sons and daughters. You may have an interest in getting into a good relationship with such fathers.

Narcissistic Mother

Every person alive need validation. Most of the time, healthy parents feel as if their children directly depict their narcissistic nature. Not all children are given liberty to grow and be whoever they want to be by themselves. We have earlier looked at the effects of a narcissistic father on the child, but now we want to focus on the narcissistic father and its impact on the children. Validation is an essential facet as far child nurturing is concerned. The absence or presence of a guarantee has a tremendous effect on child enabling.

A case example is a mother holding a helpless baby in her arm and the glances that the duo throw at each other means everything to the mother's soul. And to the baby, the mother's face is the perfect mirror and references that will always be sought throughout the child's life.

Do You Have A Narcissistic Mother?

This type of mother is a winner, especially when it comes to engaging the public. Even when it comes to chart career paths and even ownership of a home and being a prosperous child is never anyone's cup of tea. Still, with the presence of a narcissistic mother, you can see the impossibility becoming possible.

It is the type of woman everyone looks up to. Career-wise she is a lawyer, doctor, professor, teacher, and even she is the power behind the standing of your church, the epitome of balance. Balancing between family social aspects and becoming the pillar of societal expectations without apologetics for anything whatsoever.

Narcissist Child

A situation where a personality disorder becomes deeply related to one's excess love towards oneself, valuing your own opinions over the rest, then the condition is referred to as Narcissistic Personality Disorder (NDP)

Such children believe that they are superior and so should be treated differently and from the rest, and they disregard the feelings of the rest. It should not be confused with rational self-love because individual tends to have a sense of self-worthiness, but narcissist children take it too far. We can, therefore, see how an NDP child differs from the average child.

Many children are not born narcissists but rather made by the consistent pampering and making them believe they are the family's crème de la crème. It fills their minds with self-worthiness thoughts that would, then, be irreversible in adulthood. Also, narcissistic parents tend to affect their kids. When narcissistic parents see a child as a threat when they possess individuality, they tend to curb it. The child grows up and behaves the way a parent did, thinking that was the way of life. Also, negative criticism in excess makes the child feel incapacitated and inadequate and, in turn, becomes a narcissist to counter the negativity.

Adopted and children from divorced families are, most of the time, so insecure and feel they are not loved. They feel vulnerable, and so they develop a calloused attitude and them self-love to curb the inadequacy that they have. Also, the expectation from somewhat irrational parents makes the child esteem themselves too high or too low, and either of the conditions leads to Narcissism.

People who were abused in their tender age become narcissists unwittingly because they would rather avoid the world in its entirety than be with people who never see anything good in them.

Chapter 26. The Narcissistic Scale

Narcissism is not a rare trait. It is a usual trait found in people but just in variable amounts. The truth is that nearly every one of us will have a few characteristics that place us on the narcissism scale. The concept of spectrum stems and the narcissism spectrum denotes the severity of an individual's condition. You will see that narcissists tend to share self-importance attributes and a colossal ego in the range of narcissism. However, the amount of vulnerability in a person and their sense of grandiosity will tend to vary. Psychologists often use this narcissism spectrum scale to check on narcissism in a person and diagnose a narcissistic personality disorder.

The narcissism spectrum goes from 0 to 10. The lower the number, the less narcissistic a person is. The higher the number, the more narcissistic the person is. The ones in the middle tend to have a balanced amount of narcissism that is healthy. One half of the spectrum includes people who are amongst the healthy narcissists. They are realistic and have balanced traits. The soaring on the range you go, the individuals have more detrimental characteristics. They have a sense of arrogance instead of healthy self-esteem. They are more aggressive than assertive, and it can turn to capitulation. The higher the number, the more self-centered the person will be. They will have destructive behavioral traits and unhealthy thought processes. It would be best to infer that it is not acceptable to be too high or too low on this scale. The ideal placement in the spectrum is in the middle.

Let's look at the different numbers on the scale and what they signify:

Level 0 on the spectrum is an indicator of the unhealthily low amount of narcissism. A person placed at 0 tends to be too selfless and is easily manipulated by others. They take care of others more than their own needs and will easily bow down to others. These people are perfect and humble. However, they lack self-esteem and self-love.

Level 1 on the spectrum has people who are a little better than those at 0. These people pay a bit more attention to their personal needs. However, these people are not confident in social gatherings and tend to avoid social interaction. They get overwhelmed quite easily and hence are shy. They are humble as well but have a little sense of self-esteem. Level 2 and 3 have more social individuals. These people allow themselves to have dreams and goals. They are more comfortable in social situations than those on level 0 or 1. However, these people do not like being the center of attention too often. They can get out of their comfort zone at times but usually, restrain themselves.

Level 4, 5, and 6 have people who fall in the list of healthy narcissists. These people are humble but also have a healthy amount of self-confidence. They like getting attention from others and feeling appreciated when it is due. They know when they deserve care and when they should allow others to gain recognition as well. They don't have an unhealthy need to be at the center of everything. Nor do they fall so low in the spectrum that they shy away from attention. They have a balanced amount of self-esteem and humility.

Level 7 and 8 have a little more narcissism than is healthy. They like to boast their material possessions and achievements. However, they are also willing to acknowledge when they are in the wrong and try to improve. But these people tend to go back and forth between good and bad behavior. They like attention and are not entirely stable personalities.

Level 9 has individuals who thrive on attention and praise. They are always seeking to be at the center of things. However, they do become aware of their unrealistic need for attention and praise at some point. It makes them guilty, but they still try to hide this guilt. They know it is wrong for them to seek attention all the time but cannot seem to help themselves.

Level 10 is at the end of the spectrum. It includes people who are very self-serving and arrogant. Such individuals have a superb idea of themselves, and these are the ones who are categorized under NPD. They are known to be willing to do anything to get what they want. They will comfortably lie, cheat, steal, etc. and do anything to get attention. They love showing superiority and making others feel inferior.

There are three types of unhealthy narcissists. Their personalities are not alike from each other, but they are all narcissistic in a harmful way. A common trait amongst these three types of people is that they consider themselves better and above anyone else.

Extroverted Narcissists

They are loud and obnoxious people who love attention. They are very outgoing and like being in social situations. They live to be the center of attention in any gathering. These are always posted pictures on social media and want to show off their high life and expensive purchases. They will brag till kingdom come when they achieve something.

Introverted Narcissists

They are scared of being judged by others and may avoid people because of this. They think of themselves as superior to others but don't want others to know this. They prefer their own company and revel quietly in their sense of superiority.

Communal Narcissists

They like to show that they always do for others without asking for anything in return. They want others to acknowledge that they are like saviors for people and are still giving more than they ever take.

Now you can see just how differently narcissistic people can be. You can observe yourself and the people around you to see where they fall in the narcissism spectrum. It will give you a better understanding of their personality and will help you deal with them better.

Chapter 27. Narcissism and Culture

The "Me Decade"

Were you already alive in the 1970s to 1980s? If you were, then you may have remembered how the Eighties were specially labeled as the "Me Decade," although hints of things to come were present in the Seventies. Ads were focused on the pleasure of the consumer. The consumer was – and still is - bent on getting what he wanted.

Today, ads are doing the same. "This product will make your work less." "This will make you look good than the rest." You will hear many points that support the idea of you getting better, healthier, prettier, and so on. The narcissist self is interested in improvement.

Nowadays, you will notice that there is a reemerging and strengthened narcissism in popular culture. So many narcissists are even finding themselves in positions of eminence. Why is this the case?

Celebrities

Take, for example, the most obvious: celebrities. Their lives are now even more open to the public eye. Social media enable them to reach out to a more excellent fan base. There used to be a sense of pule and sophistication in the way celebrities present themselves. You will only see them in movies or 10-minute interviews. They may pose for the cameras while entering awards shows. Today, it is a whole lot different. Celebrity expression becomes more immersive. Adulation is more pronounced whenever fans watch their reality television shows and even their live videos on social media or personal websites. It goes beyond promotion. In their narcissism, celebrities believe that their lives are so important, it should be made into a lucrative business. Perfumes are named after celebrities, not just perfume designers. Fans want to smell like their favorite stars. The examples go on and on.

Social Life/Corporate Culture

A new type of narcissism is emerging. It is the kind that is accepted and even supported. This modern concept of self-glorification is viewed as the antithesis of socialism. It strips the person of the need to be connected to the rest of society. The narcissist is not interested in brotherhood and cooperation. He is more interested in advancing himself and his necessities in this power-hungry and money-attached world. Narcissism is also beginning to be viewed in a semi-positive light. It is thought to be a means of defense against violence, rather than a perverted and extreme self-love version. Sigmund Freud even believed that narcissism is necessary. Freud is more interested in narcissism's connections to the health of the id and the ego. Compare this to Erich Fromm's readiness to take every parochial reason, especially the one that distances narcissism from socialism.

No matter what the psychoanalysts may say, narcissism is becoming harmful to the narcissists' mental states and the enablers. The example that has been mentioned a few paragraphs ago is that the celebrity is the narcissist, and the fan is the enabler. It is a potent relationship, in which the fan is immersed under the more assertive personality of the celebrity. Some fans may even dissociate and start seeing themselves as a version of their idols. They can develop their narcissism brand to cope with the fact that they are not as famous or as wealthy as they are admiring. So, yes, they may also succumb to the tempting illusion of the narcissist's world.

Psychology Versus Sociology

If you focus on narcissism's psychology, you will be looking at one individual or at least types of the same kind of individual. On the other hand, sociology is more of a study of a group or a society. This guide may look at how narcissism is becoming more acceptable in society, but the effects on each individual vary.

Sociology affects narcissism, however. Societies that promote individualism over communalism – or the individual over the collective community – are more likely to see a rise in narcissism. On the other hand, societies that promote cooperation may still have a population of narcissists, but most are more receptive to other people's needs. In contrast, a narcissist will only think of his good. Historian Cristopher Lasch blames "cultural progressivism" and "market forces" for nearly breaking the formerly tight ties among family and community members.

Self-Advancement and Self-Preservation as A Means To Survive
Today, a lot of people have to choose their survival over others. You cannot blame them for most of the time. People have to eat. People have to make sure that they survive.

Here are a few situations that you have to examine closely:

Mr. Smith works for a company that is being labeled as corrupt. This supposedly corrupt company has strong ties with the government to be closed anytime soon. There are lots of perks in this company. Other people have left the company because of their convictions and moral judgment. Some have gone on protests to fire the corrupt head. Mr. Smith is not joining any such complaint. He does not want to lose his high-paying job.

Denise posts several pictures of herself on her social media. The images all portray the same positions. Her face is usually highlighted and even filtered to look extra good. She earns money from the likes that she gets. She even gets to promote products for a fee. Friends and family advised her to find a different job because of the backlash she has been getting. Denise does not care about what other people think. She gets through life very quickly, compared to other people. She pays for her rent and other bills.

The community of Al Fresco is conducting a book drive. The book drive aims to collect as many books as possible from the families in the neighborhood. The books will be donated to public schools and to homes where books are scarce. The Peters family has heard of the book drive, but they are too busy with their busy schedules. Not one member has decided to take books from their overflowing shelves. The book drive is not their business. It does not directly affect them.

Emil is home before anyone else in the family. He takes this as an opportunity to grab the ice cream tub. There is still enough ice cream for the whole family, but Emil has declared first dibs on the entire thing. He believes that since he is the only one at home, he has the right to it. He does not care that strawberry is his sister's favorite and that she was the one who requested it from their mom.

Mrs. Shelley is a hypochondriac. Whenever her children want to go elsewhere for a vacation, she becomes sick. She will feel like throwing up. She will be dizzy. There are times that she even claims to have a fever, but she has not used a thermometer to check. She wants her children to stay with her and take care of her even if she does not have a real disease.

After reading the above, do you think any of them is a real narcissist? It can be challenging to judge with just one instance in their lives. However, you can already start guessing which ones are of the worst kind, real narcissist or not.

In the first example, Mr. Smith is only talked about based on his attitude towards work. It may just be a case of self-preservation. Self-preservation or being too focused on the self can be mistaken for narcissism. One thing is for sure: Mr. Smith will choose himself and his family over other people.

The second example may be the same thing. Denise is just working. However, there is an additional degree of selfishness and laziness involved here, as well. She does not care that other people find her superficial, and that can be a good point. However, she is not addressing her family's genuine concern: She has chosen a job with very few responsibilities and does not require a lot of skills. It will be trouble in the future.

The Peters family, in the third example, shows a lack of care and compassion for others. All they are interested in is their issues. Nothing beyond the four walls of their house can make them do something beyond what is comfortable. The Peters family may be a typical family. It may even be an ideal family. The problem here is that it is also a perfect place for raising young narcissists. The ties with the rest of the community have been cut. The children follow what their parents are doing. It has been acceptable not to care for other people when they are more than capable of extending help.

Emil, in the fourth example, may have the beginnings of a young narcissist. Maybe he considers this as pure mischief. His parents may look at it as selfishness. However, the lack of regard for other members of the family can be problematic. If not corrected by his parents, Emil may well be on his way to becoming a cold-blooded narcissist.

In the fifth and last example, Mrs. Shelley looks like an excellent example of a covert narcissist. The word "hypochondriac" is a clue here that what she has been doing is habitual. It is an example of a full-blown narcissist. However, because she looks very pitiful, she does not conform to the cultural and modern concept of what a narcissist acts and looks like. The society promotes narcissism at the level of the bossy employer, the political go-getter, the flashy celebrity, the diva singer, and so on. Even the comfort-seeking consumer is part of this growing epidemic. Mrs. Shelley is a narcissist but not of the kind that is being talked about in this guide.

Narcissism in The Modern World

There are some trends and patterns that you can observe regarding narcissism. This personality disorder is becoming more commonplace in the modern world. However, it is noticed that it is more pronounced in the Western world than in the Eastern world.

A study that can prove this is one that was conducted on both West and East Germany. The controlled research had participants from either side from the same demographics. The results showed that West Germans have greater narcissistic makeup, while East Germans have higher self-esteem. It proves that not all parts of the world are directly affected by the narcissism epidemic. West and East Germany do not even belong to different parts of the world. They are parts of a whole. However, there is a different mindset in one that affects the population of narcissistic people.

At that point, you may start questioning some of the traits that this modern society has gifted you. Is it a blessing or a curse? The paradox here is that the community that you are supposed to be actively participating in and cooperating with maybe the thing that provides you with the ammunition to become selfish and self-absorbed. The examples that you see from celebrities and other famous people may be the ones that introduce you to your narcissistic self. After all, why can't you be like the movie stars, the published writers, the wealthy footballers, and the fluent politicians? Aren't what they are showing recipes for success? And don't you want to have some of that?

Chapter 28. Dissecting the Workaholic Narcissist

Giving You the Benefit

As children, we were taught to give people the benefit of the doubt. In other words, if someone takes a deliberate action against you and hurts your feelings, excuse them for it, even if you believe they had bad intentions. We were taught to give people many chances to mistreat us and forgive them for it. It can also mean to decide to believe someone, even if you're not sure that what the person is saying is true. It means to assume a person is innocent until it can be proven otherwise.

The Amazing Worst Combo

Narcissists and people with Obsessive-Compulsive Personality Disorder value and devalue others. You will often see this trait in the workaholic narcissist. It confuses their victims. When something is valued, you see it as beneficial or have a high opinion of it. When a workaholic type is loving you, they put you on a pedestal. They charm you. You aren't privy to their nasty side in which others are battling. You are lathered in extra special treatment and privileges that others only dream of experiencing. They think you're pretty or handsome; they enjoy the attention you give them; they like the way you dress and how you handle situations. They think you're fun and easy to work with, and they want how nicely you treat them. You are cooperative, and you share things with them, including aspects of your job, so they don't have to struggle to invent necessary tasks. Instead, they can use what you have.

When someone with obsessive-compulsive personality disorder values you, it's because you're capable of fulfilling many requests with the best details. You reach perfection, and you're orderly, timely, and efficient. The quality in which you do things is outstanding. You don't complain about their demanding ways of doing things; you go along with it and go to extra lengths to do something with the germfree precision that some of them with OCD traits expect.

The workaholic narcissist will tell you that they don't have enough certificates to thank you for all you do for the company. To stay in their good graces, you perform at a rigid and high level, keep up with the impossible workloads thrown at you, do not complain, and are a yes ma'am, yes sir type of person. Some of them make decisions based on who dresses well and toss out applicants who do not. When they value you, you may be miserable because the expected amount of work is unrealistic. You pay the cost by having less time to rejuvenate and spend with family and friends, but the upside is that their hateful comments and negative ways are not torturing you.

When the workaholic type likes someone, they intuitively know they need to walk on eggshells to stay in good graces. Once they are hated, the wrath that comes with their sudden shift can make one's life miserable. The workaholic narcissist splits, so they value and devalue, meaning that their defense mechanisms allow them to put people in one category or the other. You can't be in both classes simultaneously, meaning there's no room for human error. You are either excellent or the worst. Remember, this is someone who more than likely experienced abuse in which they had to learn to make quick judgments about people for mere survival. Although this helped them survive in childhood, the people who are not abusing them pay for the crime of those who did because they didn't learn to make differences between those who are abusive and those with good intentions. Everyone will be placed in the same barrel, offensive or not.

The Villain and Superman Unite

Let's examine the workaholic type in terms of the id, ego, and superego. These three Freudian terms make up the psyche. The id is the part within us that functions on what's instinctual and is the undercurrent of who we are. It pertains to areas like aggression, hidden memories, reveals itself in dreams, and represents our aggressive and sexual drives. The superego is the moral compass that questions ethics and values. It is the part of us that creates guilt to make us do the right thing and guides us to make conscientious decisions. The ego is the middleman. It serves as the conscious and represents reality, balance, and regulates our lives. Can you guess which constructs are operating in overdrive in the NPD and the OCPD? The Narcissistic Personality Disorder operates in excessive id mode while the Obsessive-Compulsive Personality Disorder is functioning in extreme superego mode.

Picture the workaholic narcissist who is trying to satisfy two personality disorders simultaneously. Housed inside one person is the superego fighting for the extreme left while the id fights for the extreme right. Imagine how hard the brain must work to execute requests that come from excessive dual degrees. Imagine the internal confusion that the person experiences while struggling to satisfy each personality disorder. Not only that, but these people often disseminate confusing messages to the people around them that don't make sense. That's because various parts of the brain are in overdrive at the same time. The workaholic type can have a flood of internal confusion that interferes with decision-making, which is why they may let someone else step up in certain areas or divvy out particular tasks. They are scattered when it comes to the orders they give, which makes some employees angry that they're not allowed to play a role in which they were hired.

Under the Haze of COVID-19

Remember the coronavirus outbreak in 2020? By early March, the United States had its first outbreak. The virus rapidly spread as the US tried to slow the virus down by quarantining everyone. Businesses closed, and the Nation's schoolchildren were instructed to stay home indefinitely and use technology to communicate with teachers and receive classwork. Parents were now homeschooling. Churches closed, and thanks to technology like Facebook Live and YouTube, they could broadcast from home. The goal was not to reach a peak that the medical system could not handle. Slow and steady for the growth of the highly contagious novel illness was the plan so that health care workers could adequately care for patients and have enough equipment to save lives. People were instructed to wash their hands frequently for twenty seconds. Avoid touching one's face, practice social distancing by remaining six feet apart and stay as close to their clean, safe home as possible.

During the time of quarantine, workaholic narcissists struggled too, but in different ways. Hard to satisfy, how would they react now that holes were poked in their narcissistic supply tank? They quickly shifted gears, probably quicker than most people pouncing immediately on coworkers, by first exploiting group chats. People politely asked them to back off to figure out their priorities and how to proceed, but the workaholic types ignored their pleas and kept piling on their drummed-up ideas and visions. Nervous, they couldn't risk losing any "bottom-dwellers" and acted quickly to reestablish connections and invent tactics to build new suppliers. How could they make themselves needed in this new arena? Determined to infiltrate the game before they faded into nothing-land, they eagerly ambushed people's weaknesses. They sought opportunities to protrude their chests and make others feel feeble compared to their high intelligence. They immediately showed how quickly they could grasp new skills in the middle of a storm, sometimes making uncaring, thoughtless decisions that only served to fatten their pocketbooks.

OCPD narcissists are hard to satisfy. Narcissistic supply tank drips empty all the time, so during the COVID-19 outbreak, their mission was to build up an "at the home network" to be fed. They conjured up ways to get compliments, have power over others—a double-edged sword as they started to look at the people who needed them as highly unintelligent, which they despise. Needing the workaholic narcissist, not requiring them or not executing as quickly as they'd infuriate them. As much as they need people to feed their hunger for power, they contradict themselves. Do they want to know why they are continually being bothered? Answer: they have systematically made others depend on them. In their minds, they are brighter, smarter, and far more knowledgeable than you even when they dish out irrational ideas and demand that everyone follow suit.

You are expected to answer and report to them, even in quarantine, even if they are not your boss. They don't trust you to do your part—at least not to their standards. They control their environment by controlling you. Instead of focusing on their private shambles that warrant attention, their site is set on you to replenish their needed supply.

Picture yourself during COVID-19. If your company was told to work from home effectively immediately, how would a workaholic narcissistic boss respond? Many of them schemed, forced their associates back into the workplace unnecessarily, even when it was against policy, to potentially expose them to coronavirus. They couldn't let go of their lifeline. Panic set in. This brand of folks manipulated, finding loopholes in orders, placing their coworkers in high-risk situations, insisting and threatening that they report to the workplace. They were going to wield their power around to satisfy their own needs, regardless of whether they had elderly parents in the home, not caring if they were putting their associates' lives in jeopardy. Some people were even ordered to remove their masks and gloves. Meanwhile, no one knew which of these workers were bullied and had already had contact with COVID-19.

Contact tracing was used to inform people when they had been exposed to someone with the virus. Before permanent lockdown, one workaholic narcissist said, "When I leave the country in a couple of days, I'm not reporting back to management. It's none of their business. If I let them control this part of me, they'll try to control me in other ways too." Trying to rationalize with the person that this is an unusual circumstance is difficult. It's for the safety of all. They retort that if they get COVID-19, you're getting it too.

It is not someone innocent who desires to continue enjoying life without letting fear stop them from the pleasures of life. It is negatively rebelling against authority and not caring about how their behavior impacts others. Interestingly, we often follow the lead and seek approval from individuals with deficits in their personalities when the person with debts should be following us. People with these personality disorders are permitted to take control in ways that they are not emotionally mature enough to handle.

They want the power and don't want anyone else to have it. Even in normal circumstances, they can become belligerent when told what to do. Everyone was miserable, strained, and uncomfortable during that time in history. Flooded with anxiety and having occasional dips into the sea of depression, all suffered in some way. It was a new way of existing that was unfamiliar, uncharted, and uncertain. It could be incredibly tricky when the NPD OCPD showed no empathy; their sole mission was to get narcissistic supply.

Chapter 29. Things That Narcissistic Hate but Ordinary People Like

Now, we'll talk about some things that the narcissists hate that ordinary people love. We will also talk about what you can do if you find yourself in a relationship with somebody like this.

They Hate Holidays

the first one is that narcissists hit holidays. They hate festivities. They hate birthdays. They hate anniversaries, and they hate anything that calls for a celebration that consists of something other than recognizing their gift to the Earth. So, suppose you're in a relationship with a narcissist. In that case, they will sabotage every special occasion and use it as a weapon to make other people miserable so that they can feed their narcissist supply. Ordinarily, special events are a time for celebrations and people's time to reflect on their values and the people they love. It is a time for people to put aside their stress and their problems and focus on the essential things to them. But that is a problem for the narcissist person because they are the only thing unique in their eyes, creating pathological jealousy.

They are jealous that other people can have genuine happiness without faking it. They are envious that other people can enjoy another people's company without thinking of how they can manipulate and get something out of somebody. They are jealous that people know how to have fun. So, when you are in this situation, you need to recognize that it is the way they are. If every year you're hoping for a different kind of anniversary or another type of special occasion that that year that things are going to be different, especially if the month before the celebration, the narcissist starts acting as if things are going to be different then you are putting yourself up to be hurt

It doesn't mean that you have to adapt to the mystery that the narcissist is hoping you do. So, look for ways to enjoy the things that you want to enjoy.

They Hate Happiness

Anytime that you are happy, they will try to stamp it out. And to explain this, think of somebody in New York City that sees a cockroach and then they grab something and slams the cockroaches to kill it. That is the way the narcissist feels when they see you or a family member being happy. Their goal is for you to be satisfied so that they will stamp it out. They are not ordinary people; they are dysfunctional; they have a distorted view of reality and themselves. So, happiness in somebody else is a threat to their false image and a threat to who they think they are. Because narcissist doesn't feel pleasure.

They tend to imitate or mirror those qualities from other people, but it is not a general authentic emotion that they are just replicating them or fabricating them. They see you as an authentic being. You have something that they will never have, and that is the ability to feel genuine happiness from your core, not from the side or something that is fabricated, but something that is reality. So that makes you better than them, and they can't take that. They need to stamp you and see you being miserable to say that they are not sad and happy. And anytime you are delighted, their reality is threatened, so that is why they hate it. Let go of what you can't control. They are not happy with what you do. But they seemed delighted at one time in the beginning, that it is just something wrong with you, and you keep on striving to get back to the get the point whereby they can find happiness in you or they can be happy when you're happy.

The narcissist hates happiness and a way for you to see that is to analyses when the fight does come about and what makes them angry. The narcissist is never angry when you are upset about something; they are always mad when everything seems fair. You think you're having a good time, you're having a great conversation with them, and the following minute they are attacking you verbally. You're on the way to a beautiful event, and you guys will start having a crazy argument that makes no sense. It is because the narcissist tries to do something to tone down your happiness. They are trying to do something to put your happiness to little. So, you have to recognize that your happiness is not dependent on them being happy with you.

It is a tough to swallow because most of us need approval from our significant other because maybe there was a wound inside us placed inside us as a child, and we feel that our worth is placed on what other people think of us. And now the person that is thinking of that is not thinking of us very positively. Hence, it puts Lemon on our wound, and we need to heal that wound to become happy and recognize that we can feel good about ourselves even if the other person chooses not to see any good in us.

They Hate Passions

You should have some key phrases if they attack your happiness. If you are enjoying something of a passion and they come and criticize it. Rather than trying to explain or making them see through your eyes, you should use a simple phrase, "like you are allowed to have your opinion, or you are allowed to see it that way, and that is ok," and it will help you to continue to be happy with the things that make you happy. Don't wipe out your happiness just because you are in a relationship with somebody that hates what ordinary people love. A narcissist is not like a familiar person. They hate when their significant other looks good. Regular people love that people find their significant other attractive or in shape. If you tell an average person that your husband is in shape and looks good, the ordinary person will say, "thank you. I'm feeling good" that is normal and realizes that their spouse looks good, but not a narcissist.

If somebody compliments their significant other, that is a threat to them because somehow, they raised their significant other and lowers them. Everything is a competition to them. Everything is measured with them. So, they hate when their significant other looks good, and that is why they try to sabotage anything good to that significant other. If their significant other is skinny, they tell them that they are too thin and need to gain weight, but they will say that they are overweight and not as attractive as they used to be when they gain weight. If you chase after trying to make them happy, you will find out that nothing you do to will make them happy, and there is no perfect weight and no perfect anything because they don't even want you to look good. They want the center to be on them.

So, focus a little bit on yourself and focus on what is more important to you. Is exercise important to you? Are you living with what is important to you? Are you making time for things that are important to you, or have you stopped doing them because somebody else doesn't like them? You need to recognize it and take small steps to get back and start doing the important things; otherwise, you will be allowing somebody to erase you just because your passions threaten their false reality. And other things that narcissists hate that ordinary people love when their significant other or family member is successful.

So now, what do you do? You have to recognize that you can't trust what a narcissist says. If they feel that you are empowering yourself, you are stepping back and trying to protect yourself. Whatever you're accomplishing in life, they will switch forms and try to be the most accommodating and helpful person trying to help you succeed. So, please don't fall for it again.

Hate When Your Kids Love You

now narcissist height when your children I love you. They hate the fact that your children enjoy being with you. Ordinary people love that the children have a relationship with the other parent. Often, it's a blessing because when your children are with the other parents, you know that they are safe, and you have some time to focus on the things you need to focus on. Because parenting is a tag team and you do things together, and the children need both parents, a narcissist will tell everybody that is the way they view it, but the truth is that they hate the fact that they want to spend time with you.

If you guys are divorced and separated and the children are on visitation, they will be punished anytime they desire to call the other parents. Or if they express that they miss the other parents, they will be punished. However, if they express anger towards the other parents, they will be well rewarded because the narcissist hates to see that the children love the other parents. Everything is a competition for them. So, if you are in this situation, you need to be aware of this.

You have to see it and recognize where it's coming from and start strategizing on to help your children view family life healthily and view their parents healthily. If they don't realize that, the children will be taught the dysfunction of the other parent. Now it is hard because if you are in a relationship with a narcissist, your head is not where it used to be, and you have been manipulated for a long time, and you can't even function as an adult to talk of helping small children. However, they need your help, or otherwise, they will grow up and think that all these things are every day. So, these are the things that narcissists hate that ordinary people love.

Conclusion

A healthy life with a narcissist is impossible. They do not know how to communicate with others in a way that is not manipulative. It is likely because as a child, they could not get their needs met by asking for them and had to go about it in an underhanded way, and as an adult, they continue this behavior. They will likely use these stories of childhood tragedies as a way of playing on your sympathy and getting you not to leave them. You can feel compassion for what they endured as a child, but you owe it to yourself not to tolerate abuse from who they have become as an adult.

It must be that a survivor does not contact the narcissist. It means they cannot share phone calls, messages, or visit this person. It will only be detrimental to their mental health and put them right back into square one. They need to keep themselves out of the risk of breaking no contact.

It means their time needs to be filled with something else so they won't have time to think about and contact the person they are trying to distance themselves from. It is the point of making new friends and reconnects with old ones. Taking up a new exciting hobby or a class will take up your time and introduce you to new people.

A person who is a victim of long-term narcissistic abuse needs some form of psychiatric care because, at this point, they are also mentally unwell. They have likely regressed into a state of learned helplessness and have cultivated a victim mentality. They do not think about what to do about their situation. They have developed a trauma bond with the narcissist, a term used to describe a victim's psychology repeatedly going back to their abuser. Partially it is because they do not think they deserve better, and they also have the idea of "it's better to live with the evil you do know than face the unknown." It is a thought process they will have to break out of to escape the cycle of abuse.

Cognitive-behavioral therapy, also known as CBT, is highly effective in treating a person trying to recover from narcissistic abuse. A therapist who practices CBT guides their patients by taking negative thinking patterns that are destructive to one's mental health and transforming them into more positive ones.

The trauma bond is a distorted thinking pattern. The victim of narcissistic abuse has become addicted to the positively emotionally-charged cycle of their relationship with the narcissist. There are several reasons for this. The constant putdowns have torn down their self-esteem. The narcissist also knows exactly how much abuse their victim can take and when they have to use the love-bombing tactics again. A narcissist might have raised the victim, so they are subconsciously gravitating toward what is familiar to them.

The person must take up a hobby where they will do something productive and meet new people. Their past abuser's insults have become the voice in their head, and this voice needs to be eliminated. For example, if they take up a sewing class, they will feel a sense of accomplishment when they have created a piece of clothing, which will automatically give them a boost in their self-esteem. They also will develop friendships with people who think well of them and show them affection.

Their kind words will eventually challenge the ones from their abuser, and ultimately, the thought will cross the person's mind- "should I listen to one person who doesn't like me, or all of these other people who do?" You have to make sure you are genuinely willing to commit to going no contact with the narcissist and everything that entails. That means blocking them on any media you could contact them through, ignoring the barrage of calls and messages that will soon follow, your urges to contact them again. The smear campaign that so many narcissists throw upon their victims when they attempt to leave them.

A covert narcissist is exceptionally skilled at starting a smear campaign. They have carefully crafted an image of themselves of being a helpless victim, and they enjoy assassinating someone else's character. The narcissist will tell others they do not know you as well as they think they do. They will try to convince everyone you are mentally unstable while masking their mental instability, driving them to do this to another person. If you remain unresponsive, everyone will see you being calm and collected while they are ranting and raving about you. Eventually, no one will want to hear them talk about you anymore.

It is a good idea to connect with people who have shared your experiences. There are online support groups for people who have been through narcissistic abuse. You will know what to expect and have support in dealing with it. There is a caveat. You need to find the right group. The right group will hold you accountable and talk you out of making mistakes like breaking no contact. They will not excuse you. A support group's goal should be to help one another move on, not stay in the same unhappy place.

If you must talk to the person because of children, work, or some other reason, use the tactic known as gray rocking. This technique has this name because the goal is to be as emotionless and uninteresting as a gray rock. Stick entirely to the facts and what needs to be done. Do not respond to anything else.

If you try to break free from their manipulation, narcissistic abuse will become a subject in your life that no longer exists, and you can pursue a life you enjoy and deserve to have.

CPSIA information can be obtained
at www.ICGtesting.com
Printed in the USA
BVHW061408250221
601119BV00001B/238

9 781802 082951